D0994791

Psychiatric Rehabilitation

Psychiatric Rehabilitation

A practical guide

Mounir Y. Ekdawi MB, ChB, DPM, FRCPsych

Consultant Psychiatrist

and

Alison M. Conning MA, MPhil, PhD

Chartered Clinical Psychologist

Netherne Hospital
Surrey, UK

Jo Campling

Commissioning Editorial Consultant

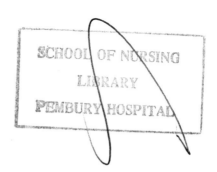

CHAPMAN & HALL
London · Glasgow · New York · Tokyo · Melbourne · Madras

Published by Chapman & Hall, 2–6 Boundary Row, London SE1 8HN

Chapman & Hall, 2–6 Boundary Row, London SE1 8HN, UK

Blackie Academic & Professional, Wester Cleddens Road, Bishopbriggs, Glasgow G64 2NZ, UK

Chapman & Hall Inc., One Penn Plaza, 41st Floor, New York NY 10119, USA

Chapman & Hall Japan, Thomson Publishing Japan, Hirakawacho Nemoto Building, 6F, 1–7–11 Hirakawa-cho, Chiyoda-ku, Tokyo 102, Japan

Chapman & Hall Australia, Thomas Nelson Australia, 102 Dodds Street, South Melbourne, Victoria 3205, Australia

Chapman & Hall India, R. Seshadri, 32 Second Main Road, CIT East, Madras 600 035, India

Distributed in the USA and Canada by Singular Publishing Group Inc., 4284 41st Street, San Diego, California 92105

First edition 1994

© 1994 Mounir Y. Ekdawi and Alison M. Conning

Typeset in Palatino 10/12pt by Mews Photosetting, Beckenham, Kent
Printed in Great Britain by Hartnolls Limited, Bodmin, Cornwall.

ISBN 0 412 49270 5   1 56593 128 9 (USA)

Contents

Preface

This book looks at the field of psychiatric rehabilitation from a practical point of view. It is based on clinical experience, illustrated with examples from day-to-day practice and draws on the most important research literature in this field. It will assist rehabilitation practitioners and trainees of all disciplines including psychiatrists, clinical psychologists, nurses, social workers, occupational therapists and health service managers, and will be a valuable source of information to students sitting professional exams.

All aspects of psychiatric rehabilitation are examined, including theoretical principles and guiding philosophies, the people involved in rehabilitation, assessment and intervention, the nature of sheltered environments used in rehabilitation and issues of resettlement and organization of services. Psychiatric rehabilitation is discussed in the context of the up-to-date and complex issue of moving from hospital-based care to care in the community; planning for individual patients; and planning services. In a world of increasing accountability, the difficult topic of outcome indicators is addressed.

As the first author is a psychiatrist and the second a clinical psychologist, the book offers an interdisciplinary account of psychiatric rehabilitation and draws on the knowledge base of both these professions.

The authors acknowledge their debt to the research and practical experience based on the work of the Netherne Rehabilitation Service. They are grateful to Sue Cook, who typed the manuscript and Dr Conning is grateful to Dr Len Rowland for comments on her manuscript.

People involved with psychiatric rehabilitation services

1

Psychiatric disability does not only affect the disabled person; it also has major consequences for the family and for others involved in the provision of long-term care and rehabilitation. For this reason, rehabilitation has been considered to be a joint venture undertaken between the disabled person and his/her helpers (Morgan and Cheadle, 1981). This chapter deals with aspects of psychiatric disability which have a bearing upon the disabled individual, the family and the staff involved in the rehabilitation process.

1.1 PEOPLE WITH PSYCHIATRIC DISABILITY

Specialized clinical services are identified by their expressed aims, by the models of care they adopt and by the interventions they use to achieve their objectives; most importantly, they are defined by the particular populations they serve. It is therefore pertinent to consider the characteristics of people severely disabled by chronic mental illness, with whom rehabilitation services are concerned (Royal College of Psychiatrists, 1987). According to a British estimate, 1.39 per 1000 of the population constitute a high-dependency disabled group, requiring high levels of long-term day care (Wing, 1982) – a modest figure compared with American estimates (Goldman, 1984). Much professional effort and time have been devoted to the nomenclature of this group (Lavender and Holloway, 1988). Terms such as 'clients', 'users', 'residents' and 'workers' have been variously used in order to avoid stigmatizing labels; these terms, however, often reflect the ideologies of different professional groups, which further complicates an already complex issue (Bachrach, 1990). The same person, nevertheless, may engage in a variety of social roles which attract particular designations – being, for example, a social worker's client, a psychiatrist's patient, a hostel resident, a user of state benefits and a worker in a sheltered factory; a single, exclusive label is neither adequate nor realistic. In these chapters, therefore, various terms will be used according to the relevant context.

1.1.1 CHRONIC MENTAL ILLNESS

The attributes of chronic mental illness have major implications in delineating the responsibilities and the management and planning arrangements of rehabilitation services, and in shaping their provisions (Ekdawi, 1990). Chronicity is defined by diagnosis (usually of functional psychosis), severity of illness and its duration (Bachrach, 1988); long-term duration is the main component of the definition. In a classical review, Brown (1960) equated chronicity with continuous hospital stay of 2 or more years; this temporal dimension was used as a reliable measure for two decades. The deinstitutionalization movement, with its trends of avoiding hospitalization whenever possible and of limiting hospital stay to a minimum, resulted in a massive reduction of hospital long-stay populations, so that only 3–5% of patients with chronic mental illness spend more than a year in hospital (Jakubaschk and Kopp, 1989). As a result, this measure has gradually been abandoned in favour of calculating duration from the time of onset of illness, rather than from the date of hospital admission. This is often inaccurate, since many serious psychiatric disorders which result in disability have an ill-defined, insidious onset. A compromise was reached whereby prolonged or repeated hospitalization was included in the indicators of chronicity, while taking into account the approximate duration of the illness. An operational definition by the National Institute of Mental Health (1977) stipulated 'a single episode of hospitalization, in the last 5 years, of at least 6 months' duration, or two or more hospitalizations within a 12-month period'. This was criticized by Goldman (1984), since it could include non-chronic conditions which might have required two brief admissions and it excluded chronic patients kept out of hospital. Despite its shortcomings, however, this imperfect yardstick continues to be used (Black, Guthrie and Bridges, 1990).

1.1.2 PATTERNS OF HOSPITALIZATION

Admission to and length of stay in hospital are determined by a variety of clinical and social factors and are influenced by the type and degree of disability; hospitalization patterns have important implications for rehabilitation provisions. Long-term hospital residents have been divided into 'old' and 'new' long-stay patients; 'old' long-stay patients were those whose period of hospitalization exceeded 5 years whereas the 'new' long-stay group was deemed to consist of those who were continuously resident for periods of 1–5 years (Department of Health and Social Security, 1971). The definition of the 'new' long-stay patients was narrowed by Mann and Cree (1976) to include those aged 15–64 years at the time of their admission whose length of stay was from 1–3 years; this was because older patients presented different problems from younger ones, and in view of changing hospital admission and discharge policies. The survey analysed the characteristics of the 'new' long-stay group and concluded that although they were so disabled that only a third could be discharged even if suitable community accommodation was available, it was far from homogenous. In the large-scale prospective Scandinavian studies, Kastrup (1987a, 1987b) highlighted the differences between patients who had histories of prolonged hospital stay and those who developed a pattern of 'revolving door' admissions; these differences were predominantly socially determined, so that the latter group tended to be drawn from younger, single or divorced city dwellers.

There is an increasing number of disabled people who, until the 1950s, would have been continuously hospitalized for many years but who are now either never admitted to hospital or, alternatively, have brief multiple admissions. Despite their severe disabilities, some have minimal or no contact with psychiatric services (Layton, 1987).

1.1.3 CLINICAL AND SOCIAL CHARACTERISTICS

The large miscellaneous group of people with chronic mental illness shows an enormously wide range of characteristics. Thus, McCreadie, Robinson and Wilson (1984) describe their typical chronic patient as a male who retains residual, mainly negative, schizophrenic symptoms; he lives alone or with aged parents and he has no obvious difficulties in personal relationships and social functioning. Bigelow et al. (1988), on the other hand, identified a younger group, mainly of chronic schizophrenic patients, with medical and/or substance abuse problems; they are socially isolated, have few self-care skills, comply poorly with treatment and show unpredictable and assaultative behaviour. In addition, other studies have shown that such young-adult chronic patients tend to be highly mobile, thus presenting further challenges to the services (Bachrach, 1982).

Chronic patients have been categorized according to their dependency levels (Wing and Furlong, 1986). The degree of independence that can be achieved by them is often complicated by several factors: risk of harm to self and others; unpredictable behaviour and liability to relapse; poor motivation and impaired capacity for self-management and for the performance of social roles; lack of insight; and low public acceptability. Wide variations in the levels of clinical and social disabilities have been reported in many other studies; there is, for instance, a group of chronic patients described by Klerman (1977) as being 'better but not well', who may manage to live in community settings but who manifest clinical, social and vocational problems (Searight and Handal, 1986). At the other end of the spectrum, Ford, Goddard and Lansdallwelfare (1987) distinguished an older, long-stay group who were extremely socially and psychiatrically disabled and who continue to need such services as are generally only provided in hospital.

In summary, the population of the chronically mentally ill, while consisting of people who have in common a combination of long-term clinical and social disabilities, is a highly heterogeneous one. There are therefore wide variations in clinical presentations and social functioning and dependency levels, as well as in patterns of hospitalization and contact with services. This has obvious implications for the provision of rehabilitation services, and in planning chains of different facilities for this population.

1.1.4 THE EXPERIENCE OF DISABILITY

The concept of social disablement includes three main elements: psychiatric impairment (or symptoms), social disadvantage and personal reactions to impairment and disadvantage (Wing and Morris, 1981). Although these personal reactions have powerful effects on the outcome of rehabilitation, subjective experiences of illness and its social implications are not always seriously considered and taken into account. This may be due to the notion that psychiatric illness invariably affects judgement and insight, but it may also be influenced by the fact that patients' first-hand experiences do not usually accord with clinical terminology, being shaped by personal factors and modified by the process of subjecting highly unusual expriences to the constraints of common language (Ekdawi, 1982). However, assessments which only focus on symptoms and social functioning levels are incomplete since they ignore the interaction between the individual and the disorder in the process of adaptation to long-term illness and disability (Strauss, 1989). Patients' accounts have greatly added to our understanding of the impact of symptoms on social performance, and how it feels to be on the receiving end of treatment, to be unemployed and to be given state benefits; some have also contributed to the clarification of certain contentious issues such as the implications of labelling for the person concerned (Mosher and Menn, 1978). In a series of essays by seven intelligent and literate patients, the authors vividly portrayed their experience of symptoms, the impact of disability on their lives in a variety of situations, their views of treatment and their striving towards adjustment (Anonymous, 1980). Another clear account by Leete (1989) lists a variety of mechanisms which she uses in coping with and managing her illness and its social consequences. These include the structuring of a predictable daily schedule of work and leisure, socializing with others who have similar problems, dealing with paranoid feelings and overcoming difficulties caused by poor concentration, and building on small successes; she also outlines methods which she found useful in decreasing environmental stresses and in conquering feelings of stigma. An understanding of these personal feelings and reactions can assist in cementing the alliance between the disabled person and the professionals, and an appreciation of these coping strategies can often be generalized to inform good rehabilitation practices.

1.2 THE RELATIVES

Family life has been considered to be one of the most powerful environmental forces which affect the course of severe mental illness, and professional views of the nature of family influences have evolved and changed over the years. At one time, families were sometimes judged to be causative agents of mental illness; work in this field tended to focus on three main aspects: relationships among family members, the content of family communications and their style. The view that abnormal family relationships were central aetiological factors was exemplified by the work of Lidz *et al.* (1958) who ascribed the incidence of schizophrenia in sons and daughters to marital skew and marital schism respectively. Abnormalities in the content of parental communications were, in the opinion of Bateson *et al.* (1956), responsible for the genesis of schizophrenia, while abnormalities of the form and style of communications were emphasized by Singer and Wynne (1965) as instrumental in causing some symptoms. A good deal of criticism was levelled at much of this work; Hirsch and Leff (1971), for instance, could not entirely replicate Singer and Wynne's results and, at the same time, pointed out that behaviours observed in families of schizophrenic patients were not unique to them. Most of these studies were criticized because the reported abnormalities could, in any case, have been the result and not the cause of illness (Mendick and McNeil, 1968).

Prior family relationships could have a significant effect on the patient's rehabilitation and resettlement once the illness becomes established (Clausen and Yarrow, 1955). More importantly, the quality of the prevalent emotional expression in the family could determine the likelihood of relapse and hospital readmission (Brown, Birley and Wing, 1972). The role of expressed emotion as a precipitant of relapse in schizophrenia has been well documented, notably by Leff and Vaughan (1985), and there has been gradual acceptance that while the family may not be the cause of illness, it could be a factor contributing to symptom relapse. There has therefore been a shift in the professional view of the family, from seeing it as pathogenic to seeing it as relapsogenic.

Family attitudes and expectations have been shown to have a relationship to the long-term outcome of rehabilitation. The patterns of family expectations depend on a variety of factors: in general, higher levels of social performance are expected from a patient with a recognized key role, for example as the main wage earner (Lefton *et al.*, 1962) and in middle class families (Freeman and Simmons, 1963). Moreover, there may exist wide differences in the interpretation of the rights and obligations attached to the patient's sick role by individual members of a family (Gordon, 1966) and in the degree of their willingness to tolerate some deviant behaviours (Mechanic, 1962). In general, however, behaviours commonly associated with the negative symptoms of schizophrenia often strain the coping abilities of the family as a whole (Kuipers and Bebbington, 1987). There has been an increasing recognition that relatives could be a positive resource in the management of patients when given the opportunity of information, training and support by the psychiatric services (Kuipers and Bebbington, 1985).

In the process of rehabilitating the image of the family, however, it should be remembered that family systems and the quality of their atmosphere change and fluctuate over time. It is therefore debatable whether one-off interventions can remain effective indefinitely.

1.2.1 SOCIAL DISABLEMENT AND THE FAMILY

As a result of deinstitutionalization and community care policies, families are expected to play a major role in the care and rehabilitation of their disabled relatives and, indeed, many provide the kinds of helpful and supportive environment which are associated with good outcome and low relapse rates. The enormity of this task can only be appreciated if the diversity of problems posed by the range of disability is borne in mind. In a study by Gibbons *et al.* (1984), relatives reported disturbed behaviour in 65% and restricted social performance in 78% of the patients living with them. Moreover, there was evidence of ill-health and problems in children in 90% of the households. Other surveys have shown that relatives find it particularly difficult to cope with the patients' disturbed behaviour, their poor communication skills, their inactivity and their excessive smoking. The unpredictability of the patients' behaviour is another source of discomfort and distress for relatives who do not know 'how to play it'. Nevertheless, in a study of 125 families, Doll (1976) found that their members cared for the patients, often without shame or distress, despite the heavy social and emotional strains, in situations which could be confusing and distressing; they also often understate the degree of hardship they experience (Fadden, Bebbington and Kuipers, 1987). Indeed, relatives have to cope with the same problems encountered by the staff of residential homes and day units, but without the benefit of professional training or of being able to call on the assistance of other staff, and often without any prospect of going off duty (Creer, Sturt and Wykes, 1982). That families are as much victims of mental illness as the patients becomes clearly evident when they are given the opportunity of group discussions (Ekdawi, 1981).

The family's emotional experience, often under conditions of duress and oppression, has been termed the 'subjective burden', while the economic and health costs, as well as the social disruption to the family constitute the 'objective burden' (Hoenig and Hamilton, 1969). The resultant picture of depression, apathy and social withdrawal, coupled with feelings of guilt and futility, can be seen in some parents (Wender et al., 1971). Similar findings are reported by Stevens (1972) in those elderly parents towards whom schizophrenic patients showed a high degree of dependence; however, she also found that some relatives saw advantages in this situation, including companionship and help with household chores. A pathological equilibrium whereby some families achieve stable, though maladaptive, adjustments through undue self-sacrifice or apathetic disengagement may result (MacCarthy et al., 1989). This equilibrium, however, is often modified by the passage of time; relatives' attitudes may oscillate from being tolerant and accepting to being critical and rejecting. Indeed, a complex amalgam of attitudes may exist so that a parent who expresses bitter disappointment may, at the same time, be thankful for small mercies.

Many disabled people rely on the relatives with whom they live for many of their social activities (see also Chapter 5), and they are often less able to shed the attributes of the sick role than some who live away from their families. Although families may provide a protected, helpful and undemanding environment, this can contribute to the patients' social helplessness; the strikingly low level of expectations set by some families, based on past experience of false hopes and disappointments, can de-skill and further handicap the patients and undermine their confidence. This, in turn, reinforces the relatives' persistent fears for the patients' future when they are no longer around.

In conclusion, various studies have pointed to the presence of a strong association between the family's structure and its functioning and long-term mental illness. The weight of evidence is that this association is correlational and not definitely aetiological. The patterns of family burden and coping strategies which result from the disability of one of its members may well result in increase in the patients' morbidity and maladaptive behaviour, which further augments the burden.

There is good evidence that supportive family interventions could reverse this pathological cycle (Falloon *et al.*, 1985; Kuipers and Liberman, 1986; MacCarthy *et al.*, 1989), thus enhancing the family's role within the care team as a valuable rehabilitation resource. However, the relationship between relatives and professional staff does not always run smoothly; instead of being a mutually helpful partnership, it is sometimes characterized by poor communication, hostility and suspicion or, alternatively, by excessive dependency and demandingness (Birley and Hudson, 1983). Some families who apparently need most help may receive very little; interventions and other supports which could have positive effects are denied them because of the predilection of some of the staff to devote much time to some 'rewarding' families while writing off some others as unworkable (Spitzer, Morgan and Swanson, 1972). Relatives often view the professional staff as unhelpful or indifferent to their needs, and feel that the staff blame the family for the patient's illness and disability (Willis, 1982); interviews with 56 family members indicated a high level of dissatisfaction with the services. The analysis of this sample also revealed that parents were significantly more satisfied with the service than spouses, siblings or children and that men were more satisfied than women; the level of satisfaction rose with time. The most significant factor in increasing relatives' satisfaction was supportive interaction with the service's staff representatives. Relatives' support groups, in addition to providing this type of interaction, are an excellent medium for mutual support (Ekdawi, 1981).

1.3 OTHER CARERS – THE REHABILITATION TEAM

The provision of essential facilities, such as housing and day units, is not necessarily a guarantee of the adequacy of a rehabilitation service; the most important resource in a service is its staff (Simms, 1981). It has been observed that relatives caring for a disabled family member have to acquire a diversity of skills associated with the roles of nurses, social workers and occupational therapists (Wing and Creer, 1980); they also have the advantages of first-hand experience, through trial and error, which may facilitate the creation of suitable environments, including optimal levels of social stimulation, as well as continuity of care. It may not be too fanciful to argue that other carers, professional and voluntary, should learn to perform the role of surrogate relatives; this would enhance their practical skills, by building on their theoretical knowledge, without running the risk of being too emotionally involved. Relatives have little choice in whom they should look after and they cannot impose selection criteria; other carers may also learn from them not to be too selective, thus excluding many disabled people from help on the grounds that they are not suitable for rehabilitation.

1.3.1 THE TEAM

There is ample literature on the composition of rehabilitation teams. In general, they comprise a core group of nurses, doctors, clinical psychologists and occupational therapists, with input from others including employment coordinators, physiotherapists, teachers and volunteers. The various specialist contributions are described by many authors, for example Simms (1981) and the Richmond Fellowship (1983). The wide spectrum of clinical and social problems presented by each disabled individual demands a co-ordinated input from members of many disciplines (Ekdawi, 1990) and each discipline, with its specific educational and ideological background, can actively contribute to rehabilitation programmes.

Working with disabled people is highly rewarding and intellectually challenging; it is also demanding and may be stressful. Although the acquisition of specialized knowledge and training by carers is vital (Goering et al., 1989), it should be remembered that the most highly qualified are not necessarily the most effective, since the translation of academic knowledge into practical work is a prerequisite for the management of disability. Job satisfaction in rehabilitation is often largely dependent on the carer's personal qualities, which should include energy, a pragmatic outlook and a low frustration threshold, combined with the ability to persevere and to take a long-term view rather than to seek gratification from quick results. Dissatisfaction and burn-out could result from a variety of factors, and some of these issues will now be considered.

A common cause of frustration is the occasional lack of a conceptual framework for rehabilitation work and the absence of shared clear service goals. A common vision enables the team to cope more effectively with the difficult behaviours presented by some disabled people, the fluctuations of their functioning and the occasional unpredictable deterioration and lack of 'progress'; these features are often encountered in the rehabilitation of the long-term mentally ill and they may be construed by some carers as evidence of failure, to which they may react by feeling guilty and disillusioned or by becoming hostile towards the rehabilitee. Even unforeseen improvement, leading to increased activity, autonomy and assertiveness instead of inactivity and docility, could be perceived by the carers as signs of relapse or acting out, requiring remedial action (Mason, Gingrich and Siris, 1990).

Since rehabilitation is a multidisciplinary endeavour, problems within the team may arise from uncertainties about the specific roles of its different members. This is compounded by the fact that some overlap in these roles is inevitable and that some functions have to be shared, as well as by the diversity of professional training backgrounds and value systems which, in turn, may lead to rivalries and misunderstandings. Long-term care is the sum total of negotiations, rules and agreements amongst those working in partnership, and it is therefore imperative in team work to clarify common goals and to agree on day-to-day practices (Freudenberg, 1966). Different professional roles are neither rigid nor static; they undergo modifications over time, often in response to changes in training policies or in provision, for example, from staff being anchored to a hospital base to working in multiple community settings. This means that team members need to keep abreast with developments within the various disciplines and to adapt to these changes.

Difficulties may also arise between the rehabilitation team and those working in other clinical areas. These may be due to differing professional orientations as, for instance, in the programme reported by Lang and Rio (1989) where conflict developed between psychotherapy practitioners and rehabilitation clinical teams. Other clinical areas may also harbour negative attitudes towards long-term patients, which may be reflected in similar attitudes towards rehabilitation staff and systems (Danley, Rogers and Nevas, 1989). In another example, Chant (1986) commented on the discord between some British rehabilitation services and social services departments whose organizational structures and ideological stances were so much at variance that they presented difficulties in staff working together in a meaningful way. There is a danger, in such situations, of the rehabilitation team becoming isolated and prone to collective feelings of being misunderstood and persecuted. This, in turn, may result in a less healthy culture which adversely affects the team's working efficiency.

A negative 'solution' to these problems has been a move, in some areas, towards deprofessionalization and the creation of non-specialist mental health workers, based on the erroneous belief that disabled people need only to be presented with opportunities to develop, normally, a multitude of new skills; many disabled people, however, require expert professional help to enable them to acquire appropriate behavioural and social repertoires (Cullen, 1986). There is, in fact, evidence that the performance of non-professional staff improves when they become, to some extent, professionalized; in a 12-year follow-up study of people providing private accommodation for chronic patients discharged from hospital, an increasing professional orientation to mental health care resulted in improved services and a better quality of life for the residents (Segal, Hazan and Kotler, 1990). This is not to argue for the conversion of voluntary services into professional organizations. Non-professional workers bring important qualities to rehabilitation services: they have valuable practical skills and common sense attitudes, and they are often in touch with local conditions; they are able to communicate with disabled people on a more every-day informal level and they are also, generally, more adaptable, having to contend with much less red tape than their professional colleagues. A balanced compromise may be the acceptance that voluntary work should be supplemented by professional input.

There are various mechanisms which are used to maintain team morale and to enhance the cohesiveness and effectiveness of the rehabilitation team. Each team member, however junior, should have opportunities to contribute to decision-making, both in the individual programmes and in administrative meetings, and to undertake specific tasks; it is also essential, in this connection, to give praise whenever a task is well performed. The career development and educational opportunities of each team member must be seen as a priority. Teaching, including that based on recent research, and encouragement to engage in research projects are crucial in maintaining interest in rehabilitation practice. Attendance at training courses, lectures and seminars can be of enormous educational value, but this should not be seen as a substitute for hands-on training; a student can learn much more from working with a patient, under supervision, and from presenting individual problems for discussion by the team. Opportunities to meet others working in the rehabilitation field, whether through visits or by attending some training meetings, may lessen the risks of stagnation and isolation. Staff support groups, where individual issues and common team concerns can be aired and resolved, are invaluable. Last, but not least, due care should be given to the organizational aspect of the team; a rehabilitation purpose and culture can be maintained only if a sufficient number of its senior members remain constant, while allowing for trainee members to move on as part of their education and development.

REFERENCES

Anonymous (1980) Schizophrenia from within, in *Coping with Schizophrenia*, (ed. H. Rollin), Andre Deutsch, London.
Bachrach, L.L. (1982) Young adult chronic patients: an analytical review of the literature. *Hospital and Community Psychiatry*, **33**, 189–197.
Bachrach, L.L. (1988) Defining chronic mental illness – a concept paper. *Hospital and Community Psychiatry*, **39**, 388.
Bachrach, L.L. (1990) What's in an adjective? or an acronym? *Hospital and Community Psychiatry*, **41**, 601.
Bateson, G., Jackson, D.D., Haley, J. and Weakland, J. (1956) Toward a communication theory of schizophrenia. *Behavioural Science*, **1**, 251–264.
Bigelow, D.A., Cutler, D.L., Moore, L.J. *et al.* (1988) Characteristics of state hospital patients who are hard to place. *Hospital and Community Psychiatry*, **39**, 181–185.
Birley, J. and Hudson, B. (1983) The family, the social network and rehabilitation, in *Theory and Practice of Psychiatric Rehabilitation*, (eds F.N. Watts and D.H. Bennett), John Wiley & Sons, Chichester.
Black, D., Guthrie, E. and Bridges, K. (1990) Careers in psychiatric specialities – 1. Rehabilitation psychiatry. *Psychiatric Bulletin*, **14**, 665–667.
Brown, G.W. (1960) Length of hospital stay and schizophrenia: a review of statistical studies. *Acta Psychiatrica Scandinavica*, **35**, 414–430.
Brown, G.W., Birley, J.L.T. and Wing, J.K. (1972) Influence of family life on the course of schizophrenic disorders: a replication. *British Journal of Psychiatry*, **121**, 241–258.
Chant, J. (1986) Making ends meet – a continuum of care, in *The Provision of Mental Health Services in Britain: The Way Ahead*, (eds G. Wilkinson and H. Freeman), Gaskell, London.
Clausen, J.A. and Yarrow, M.R. (1955) Introduction: mental illness and the family. *Journal of Social Issues*, **2**, 3–5.
Creer, C., Sturt, E. and Wykes, T. (1982) The role of the relatives, in *Long-term Community Care: Experience in a London Borough*, (ed. J.K. Wing). Psychological Medicine Monograph Supplement 2. Cambridge University Press, Cambridge.
Cullen, C. (1986) Multidisciplinary and consumer views, in *The Provision of Mental Health Services in Britain: The Way Ahead*, (eds G. Wilkinson and H. Freeman), Gaskell, London.
Danley, S.K., Rogers, S. and Nevas, D.B. (1989) A psychiatric rehabilitation approach to vocational rehabilitation, in *Psychiatric Rehabilitation Programs – Putting Theory into Practice*, (eds M.D. Farkas and W.A. Anthony), Johns Hopkins University Press, Baltimore.
Department of Health and Social Security (1971) *Census of Patients in Mental Hospitals and Units in England and Wales at the End of 1971*, HMSO, London.

Doll, W. (1976) Family coping with the mentally ill: an unanticipated problem of deinstitutionalisation. *Hospital and Community Psychiatry*, **27**, 183–185.

Ekdawi, M.Y. (1981) Counselling in rehabilitation. In: *Handbook of Psychiatric Rehabilitation Practice*, (eds J.K. Wing and B. Morris), Oxford University Press, Oxford.

Ekdawi, M.Y. (1982) Living with schizophrenic disabilities. *Postgraduate Medical Journal*, **58**, 648–652.

Ekdawi, M.Y. (1990) The components of psychiatric rehabilitation services, in *International Perspectives in Schizophrenia*, (ed. M. Weller), John Libby, London.

Fadden, G., Bebbington, P. and Kuipers, L. (1987) The burden of care: the impact of functional psychiatric illness on the patient's family. *British Journal of Psychiatry*, **150**, 285–292.

Falloon, I., Boyd, J.L., McGill, C.W. *et al.* (1985) Family management in the prevention of morbidity of schizophrenia. Clinical outcome of a two-year longitudinal study. *Archives of General Psychiatry*, **42**, 887–896.

Ford, M., Goddard, C., Lansdallwelfare, R. (1987) The dismantling of the mental hospital? Glenside Hospital surveys 1960–1985. *British Journal of Psychiatry*, **151**, 479–485.

Freeman, H.E. and Simmons, O.G. (1963) *The Mental Patient Comes Home*, John Wiley, New York.

Freudenberg, R.K. (1966) Functions and attitudes of professional staff in psychiatric hospitals. *Proceedings of the Royal Society of Medicine*, **59**, 591–594.

Gibbons, J.S., Horn, S.H., Powell, J.M. and Gibbons, J.L. (1984) Schizophrenic patients and their families – a survey in a psychiatric service based on a DGH unit. *British Journal of Psychiatry*, **144**, 70–77.

Goering, P., Huddart, C., Wasylenki, D. and Ballantyne, R. (1989) The use of rehabilitation case management to develop necessary supports: community Rehabilitation Services, Toronto, Canada, in *Psychiatric Rehabilitation Programs – Putting Theory into Practice*, (eds M.D. Farkas and W.A. Anthony), Johns Hopkins University Press, Baltimore.

Goldman, H.H. (1984) Epidemiology, in *The Chronic Mental Patient*, (ed. J.A. Talbott), Grune & Stratton, New York.

Gordon, G. (1966) *Role Therapy and Illness*. College & University Press, New Haven, C.T.

Hirsch, S.R. and Leff, J. (1971) Parental abnormalities of verbal communication and the transmission of schizophrenia. *Psychological Medicine*, **1**, 118–127.

Hoenig, J. and Hamilton, M. (1969) *The Desegregation of the Mentally Ill*. Routledge & Kegan Paul, London.

Jakubaschk, J. and Kopp, W. (1989) On characterising new psychiatric long-stay patients. *Social Psychiatry and Psychiatric Epidemiology*, **24**, 88–95.

Kastrup, M. (1987a) Prediction and profile of the long-stay population – a nation-wide cohort of first time admitted patients. *Acta Psychiatrica Scandinavica*, **76**, 71–79.

Kastrup, M. (1987b) Who becomes revolving door patients? Findings from a nation-wide cohort of first time admitted psychiatric patients. *Acta Psychiatrica Scandinavica*, **76**, 80–88.

Klerman, G. (1977) Better but not well: social and ethical issues in the deinstitutionalisation of the mentally ill. *Schizophrenia Bulletin*, **3**, 214–225.

Kuipers, L. and Bebbington, P. (1985) Relatives as a resource in the management of functional illness. *British Journal of Psychiatry*, **147**, 465–470.

Kuipers, L. and Bebbington, P. (1987) *Living with Mental Illness*. Souvenir Press, London.

Kuipers, L. and Liberman, R.P. (1986) Coping and competence as practical factors in the vulnerability – stress model of schizophrenia, in *Treatment of Schizophrenia: Family Assessment and Intervention*, (eds M.J. Goldstein, I. Hand and K. Halweg), Springer-Verlag, Berlin.

Lang, E. and Rio, J. (1989) A psychiatric rehabilitation vocational program in a private psychiatric hospital, in *Psychiatric Rehabilitation Programs – Putting Theory into Practice*, (eds M.D. Farkas and W.A. Anthony), Johns Hopkins University Press, Baltimore.

Lavender, A. and Holloway, F. (eds) (1988) Community Care in Practice, John Wiley & Sons, Chichester.

Layton, G. (1987) Community Psychiatry. *Bulletin of the Royal College of Psychiatrists*, **11**, 316.

Leete, E. (1989) How I perceive and manage my illness. *Schizophrenia Bulletin*, **15**, 197–200.

Leff, J.P. and Vaughan, C. (1985) *Expressed Emotion in Families*, Guilford Pess, London.

Lefton, M. Angrist, S. Dinitz, S. and Pasamanick, B. (1962) Social class, expectations and performance of mental patients. *American Journal of Sociology*, **58**, 79–87.

Lidz, T., Fleck, S., Cornelison, A. and Terry, D. (1958) Schizophrenia and the family. *Psychiatry*, **21**, 21–27.

MacCarthy, B., Kuipers, L., Hurry, J. *et al.* (1989) Counselling the relatives of long-term adult mentally ill: 1. Evaluation of the impact on relatives and patients. *British Journal of Psychiatry*, **154**, 768–775.

McCreadie, R.G., Robinson, A.D.T. and Wilson, A.O.A. (1984) The Scottish survey of new chronic inpatients: Two year follow-up. *British Journal of Psychiatry*, **147**, 637–640.

Mann, S.A. and Cree, W. (1976) 'New' long-stay psychiatric patients: a national survey of fifteen mental hospitals in England and Wales 1972/73. *Psychological Medicine*, **6**, 603–616.

Mason, S.E., Gingrich, S. and Siris, S.G. (1990) Patients' and caregivers' adaptation to improvement in schizophrenia. *Hospital and Community Psychiatry*, **41**, 541–544.

Mechanic, D. (1962) Some factors in identifying and defining mental illness. *Mental Hygiene*, **46**, 66–74.

Mendick, S.A. and McNeil, T.F. (1968) Current methodology in research in the aetiology of schizophrenia. *Psychogical Bulletin*, **70**, 681–693.

Morgan, R. and Cheadle, J. (1981) *Psychiatric Rehabilitation*, National Schizophrenia Fellowship, Surbiton.

Mosher, L.R. and Menn, A.Z. (1978) Enhancing psychological competence in schizphrenia: preliminary results of the Setoria Project, in *Phenomenology and the Treatment of Schizophrenia* (eds Faun, W.E., Karacan, I.,

Pokorney, A.D. and Williams, R.L.), Spectrum Publications, Jamaica, N.Y.

National Institute of Mental Health (1977) *Community Support Programme: Guidelines*. National Institute of Mental Health, Washington, DC.

Richmond Fellowship (1983) *Mental Health in the Community*, Richmond Fellowship Press, London.

Royal College of Psychiatrists (1987) Psychiatric rehabilitation updated. *Bulletin of the Royal College of Psychiatrists*, **2**, 71.

Searight, H.R. and Handal (1986) Pscyhiatric deinstitutionalisation: the possibilities and realities. *Psychological Quarterly*, **58**, 153–166.

Segal, S.P., Hazan, A.R. and Kotler, P.L. (1990) Characteristics of sheltered care facility operators in California in 1973 and 1985. *Hospital and Community Psychiatry* **41**, 1245–1248.

Simms, A. (1981) The staff and their training, In *Handbook of Psychiatric Rehabilitation Practice*, (eds J.K. Wing and B. Morris), Oxford University Press, Oxford.

Singer, M.T. and Wynne, L.C. (1965) Thought disorder and family relations of schizophrenics: IV. Results and implications. *Archives of General Psychiatry*, **12**, 201–212.

Spitzer, S.P., Morgan, P.A. and Swanson, R.M. (1971) Determinants of the psychiatric patient career, family reaction patterns and social work intervention. *Social Services Review*, **45**, 74.

Stevens, B. (1972) Dependence of schizophrenic patients on elderly relatives. *Psychological Medicine*, **2**, 17–32.

Strauss, J.S. (1989) Subjective experiences of schizophrenia: toward a new dynamic psychiatry – II. *Schizophrenia Bulletin*, **2**, 179–187.

Wender, P. Rosenthal, D., Zahn, T. and Kety, S. (1971) The psychiatric adjustment of the adopting parents of schizophrenics. *American Journal of Psychiatry*, **127**, 1013–1018.

Willis, M.J. (1982) The impact of schizophrenia on families: one mother's point of view. *Schizophrenia Bulletin*, **8**, 617–619.

Wing, J.K. (1982) Foreword, in *Long-term Community Care: Experience in a London Borough*, (ed. J.K. Wing). Psychological Medicine Monograph Supplement 2. Cambridge University Press, Cambridge.

Wing, J. and Creer, C. (1980) Schizophrenia at home, in *Coping with Schizophrenia*, (ed. H. Rollin), Burnett Books, London.

Wing, J.K. and Furlong, R. (1986) A haven for the severely disabled within the context of a comprehensive psychiatric community service. *British Journal of Psychiatry*, **149**, 449–457.

Wing, J.K. and Morris, B. (1981) Clinical basis of rehabilitation, in *Handbook of Psychiatric Rehabilitation Practice*, (eds J.K. Wing and B. Morris), Oxford University Press, Oxford.

Guiding models and philosophies

2

One of the challenges of working in psychiatric rehabilitation is that there is rarely a 'right answer', a prescribed way of intervening in a particular situation with a guaranteed degree of success. Instead, there are a number of guiding models or philosophies, with plenty of room for creativity and interpretation. These models and philosophies provide frameworks; some of the most frequently used will be examined below.

2.1 REHABILITATION: A DEFINITION

Before we begin to examine the models and philosophies which guide the process of rehabilitation, we need to be clear about what rehabilitation is. The term has been stolen by psychiatry from physical medicine, where it implies a two-stage process: (1) treating the symptoms of someone who has become physically disabled, such as by drugs and physiotherapy; and (2) then helping the person to make a relatively permanent adaptation to their environment, such as by providing ramps or a wheelchair (Bennett, 1983). Bennett (1983) discusses the evolution of the term in psychiatry, and suggests that there have been six stages in the development of the concept:

1. (a) attempting to modify an individual's psychiatric disability, then
    (b) compensating for the disability by developing other abilities and then placing the person in an environment in which these abilities can be used;
2. resettling psychiatrically disabled people in economic employment [an unrealistic and inappropriate aim for many people];
3. restoring psychiatrically disabled people to their former state, making them better, specifically by taking them out of the

psychiatric institutions [but people did not leave the asylums when they were opened, and people developed long-term psychiatric disabilities even though they had never been in hospital];

4. returning or integrating the psychiatrically disabled person into a home, school and/or work community by developing his/her skills;

5. improving the psychiatrically disabled person's capabilities and competence: an emphasis on coping not curing;

6. the process of helping the psychiatrically disabled person to make the best use of his or her residual abilities in order to function at an optimum level in as normal a social context as possible (Bennett, 1978).

Each of these stages in the development of the concept of rehabilitation has influenced, and been influenced by, the models used in rehabilitation. They will be discussed in relation to the guiding models below.

2.2 GUIDING MODELS

Why do we need guiding models? A model provides a framework for thinking about a particular issue or problem. It allows one to make hypotheses about the outcome of intervention which can be tested. If the hypotheses are not supported, then the model, and the behaviour based upon it, need to be changed. The use of a model to guide one's thinking and behaviour when intervening in rehabilitation should ensure that intervention is clearly thought through, has an explicit aim and expected outcome, and is consistent with other interventions made for the same person.

2.2.1 THE 'MEDICAL' OR CURATIVE MODEL

This model is consistent with stage 3 of Bennett's (1983) developments in the concept of rehabilitation. It has been adopted from physical medicine and in its crudest form suggests that if one observes a cluster of symptoms, one can then make a diagnosis, and that this diagnosis implies intervention in a specified way in order to produce a cure. This model does not of course fit many situations even in physical medicine, but in psychiatry its implications are detrimental. Firstly, it implies that something physical is wrong that can be treated, by doctors, with physical interventions. Whereas a physical intervention such as medication is often a very important component of an individual's care, it is only a single component, to be considered in conjunction with other interventions. Concentration solely on the physical aspects of what is wrong is not helpful, as individuals are likely to have many other aspects to their lives that influence their levels of functioning, for example the social environment and psychological factors such as self-esteem.

The medical or curative model implies that one should expect cure and that this is the only really desirable outcome (Pilling, 1991). By the time that most patients reach a rehabilitation and long-term care service, it has become obvious that their psychiatric disabilities are long-term and that all attempts to 'cure' have 'failed'. Continuing with the expectation of cure on the part of the therapist or the patient is not useful. Instead one has to aim at something closer to Bennett's fifth stage in the development of the concept of psychiatric rehabilitation: an emphasis on coping not curing; an emphasis on taking small steps towards improving functioning, while recognizing that the individual's functioning will fluctuate.

The medical or curative model also implies that the individual is sick and therefore must give up his or her normal roles and passively accept treatment. Whereas it may sometimes be useful for patients to adopt a passive sick role and come into hospital for a time during a period in which their psychiatric symptoms are exacerbated, the emphasis in rehabilitation is more usually on an active partnership with the patient, working towards improving or maintaining functioning.

On the positive side, some patients and their carers are comforted by being given a diagnosis, as it gives a reason for the symptoms and behaviour they have observed and provides reassurance that they are understood. However, the reality is that by the time most patients reach rehabilitation and long-term care services, their diagnosis predicts little about prognosis, symptoms or interventions (Summers and Hersch, 1983). Indeed, once a patient has long-term problems, knowledge of the living situation or social performance indicates more about his/her functioning than knowledge of diagnosis. It is often said that a diagnostic label placed on someone opens the door for them to be stigmatized and stereotyped. However, it is unlikely that the diagnostic label itself does this, and more likely that it comes from being known to have received treatment from psychiatric services.

2.2.2 THE DISABILITY MODEL

As implied by Bennett's sixth and current definition of rehabilitation, it is useful to think of the client of the rehabilitation service as psychiatrically disabled. Via the process of rehabilitation, disabled people are helped to adapt or readapt to their disabilities. Where a disability is permanent, the aim is to alter or adjust the environment to compensate for it (Bennett, 1978).

Wing (1978, 1981) proposed a useful model of psychiatric disability which comprises three levels:

1. primary or intrinsic impairments, which are the direct result of the 'illness', e.g. the positive symptoms (hallucinations, delusions) and negative symptoms (flatness of affect, underactivity, social withdrawal, slowness of thought and movement) of schizophrenia;
2. secondary impairments, which are not inherent features of the 'illness' but are the result of the response of significant others, such as professionals, family and public figures, to the person's 'illness' and are reflected in the individual's attitude to him or herself – the individual's attitudes will lead to such things as lack of confidence, poor self-esteem, lowered motivation, poor coping strategies and perhaps denial of the 'illness' or adoption of a sick role;
3. tertiary or extrinsic handicaps, which are disadvantages to some extent independent of the 'illness' that may nevertheless have played a role in its development or result from the primary and secondary disabilities – such things as bad housing, poverty, unemployment, poor social networks and difficult family relationships.

This three-level model is useful because it forces one to look beyond the symptoms of the 'illness', to the individual's, other people's and society's reaction to those symptoms, all of which can affect the individual's level of functioning. It also emphasizes that intervention should take place not just in the rehabilitation unit but within the broader social environment. It is applicable to patients living in any kind of setting.

Bachrach (1986b) has argued that this disability model – what she describes as 'the British view of disability' – 'permits us to focus on specific areas of need within the population and so enhances our ability to plan relevant programs'. It provides a framework which gives important clues about where to direct resources.

The disadvantages of the model are that it relies substantially on the medical model which, as we have discussed above, may not always be a useful way of conceptualizing an individual's difficulties. Although the model suggests areas of an individual's life which need to be considered, it does not indicate how one might intervene to the individual's advantage.

Wing (1978, 1981) distinguishes between disabilities (impairments) and handicaps. This distinction has been discussed by others, such as Wood and Badley (1978), who suggest that handicaps are the social and environmental consequences of disablement (cf. Wing's tertiary or extrinsic handicaps). An individual may be disabled but may or may not be handicapped by this disability. Mary may have psychiatric disabilities, but if there are a good range of opportunities for sheltered work in her area, she need not be handicapped in getting a job. The upper limit may be reached with regard to reducing an individual's disabilities, but there may be more that can be done to reduce the potential handicap suffered by the individual by changing the extrinsic factors. Handicap occurs when disabilities place the individual at a disadvantage relative to others in society and when society does not provide settings where mentally ill persons can find accommodation and compensation for their disabilities (Anthony and Liberman, 1986).

2.2.3 SKILLS MODEL

The skills model is consistent with Bennett's (1983) fourth stage in the development of the concept of rehabilitation and its refinements at the fifth stage. The skills model grew from the work of Anthony and his colleagues in the United States, who believed that

> The goal of a rehabilitation approach should be to provide the disabled person with the physical, intellectual, and emotional skills needed to live, learn, and work in the community with the least possible amount of support from agents of the helping professions. The means of achieving this goal is patient skill development, not symptom remission, and the observable measure of its achievement is change in community behaviour, not psychodynamic insights. (Anthony, 1977).

Implicit in this model is the idea that patients have lost, or have never developed skills which are essential for surviving outside psychiatric institutions, and so if one can teach them the necessary skills, then they will be able to survive. Anthony (1977) suggests a three-stage process for developing skills.

1. Identify those skill deficits that are preventing the patient from functioning effectively in his or her environments.
2. Assess the patient's present and required levels of functioning for each skill.
3. Intervene to eliminate any discrepancy between present and required level of skill by breaking the skill down into small steps, teaching the skill to the patient, allowing him or her to perform each step in an appropriate community setting, receiving feedback and differential reinforcement based on the skill performance.

More recently Anthony and his colleagues (Anthony, Cohen and Cohen, 1984; Anthony and Liberman, 1986) have suggested that patient skill development should go hand-in-hand with environmental resource development. This development in thinking has come about through the finding that, despite the evidence that patients can engage actively in skills-training procedures (Liberman, Falloon and Wallace, 1984) and learn useful skills (Anthony and Margules, 1974; Liberman *et al.*, 1986), the restoration of functioning through skills training is limited by continuing deficits and the reccurrence of symptoms. In other words, the improvements which can be brought about by skills training are much less than anticipated, and so one has to look towards changing the patient's environment to support and accommodate his or her disabilities, such as by providing sheltered work or living environments (Anthony and Liberman, 1986).

This model of rehabilitation is the basis upon which the Centre of Psychiatric Rehabilitation was founded in 1979 in Boston, USA, with Anthony as its director. Here clients are helped to set a goal which they want to achieve, to make their own choice about what it is that they are aiming for. The rehabilitation process does not begin until this choice has been made. Once the choice has been made, the support and critical skills needed by the person to achieve that goal are identified. Intervention is based on breaking the goal down into small objectives and then teaching and practising the skills, and creating the supports or resources, that the person needs to achieve these objectives (Farkas, 1990).

The advantages of the skills approach to rehabilitation are that it allows one to look at a broad range of areas of functioning, it provides individualized treatment and it uses very practical means of achieving its goals. In its modified form it does not consider the patient in isolation, but in the context of his or her environment(s) and social role(s). The disadvantages of this approach are that it does not necessarily distinguish between lacking a skill and having a skill but not using it. The reasons why a person may not be exercising a skill are therefore ignored – for example the patient may not consider the skill appropriate or relevant. The skills model also ignores the instability of the functioning of people with long-term psychiatric disabilities and assumes that progress will always be in one direction: forwards. Although it gives people hope that life can improve, the negative side of this is that failure to achieve a desired goal or skill may lead the therapist and/or client to consider themselves to have failed when in fact the goal itself may have been inappropriate. In its original form the model sees learning a skill as the only way of making up for a deficit. The modified form of the model considers environmental resources also: there may be other and more appropriate ways of achieving the same goals.

2.2.4 NEEDS MODEL

It would be easy to assume from a cursory glance at the British National Health Service and Community Care Act (Department of Health, 1990) and its consequent documents that a needs model is widely accepted both within care in the community and in the health service as a whole. For example, the first right specified in the British Patient's Charter is that every citizen has the right 'to receive health care on the basis of clinical need' (Department of Health, 1991).

Within rehabilitation and long-term care, the emphasis on meeting patients' needs has grown out of a concern to provide individualized, goal-oriented treatment based on a thorough assessment of the patient (Conning and Rowland, 1992). At the root of this concern is an eagerness to avoid those aspects of patient care associated with institutions and now known to be detrimental, such as block treatment, segregation from the outside world and depersonalization (Barton, 1959; Goffman, 1961).

Implicit in the aim of meeting patients' needs is the following assumption about process: 'if information is gathered about the patient's functioning across all areas of life, then staff will be able to identify his or her needs, and construct an individualized and appropriate treatment plan, based on the information, which will meet the identified needs' (Conning and Rowland, 1992). But cumulative evidence is now making it clear that this process is not as straight-forward as it might seem. For example, Khwaja (1985) has found that staff and patients disagree on what the patient's needs are. So whose view should one follow when deciding where to intervene? Secondly, Thapa and Rowland (1989) have found that staff and patients differ in the importance they attach to different areas of need, so mental health workers cannot assume that they know how to prioritize their patients' needs. Waismann (1988) compared the perceived needs of different groups of patients – grouped by age, sex, marital status and so on – and found that there are clear differences between such groups of patients in the importance they attach to various areas of needs, but that this was of little use in making decisions about one individual, who might belong to several groups at once. A third problem for the process of meeting patients' needs is that staff attitudes and biases about the way that patients should be cared for (that is, their attitudes towards management practices) influence the information people collect in the first place, the needs they identify and the interventions they choose (Conning and Rowland, 1992). The whole process seems to be fraught with difficulties.

As well as the apparent difficulties in the process of meeting patients' needs, there is the more fundamental problem of deciding what exactly 'needs' are. What do we mean when we talk about needs? The answer seems to be that the term 'need' is used in a variety of ways by different authors, or sometimes by the same author. For example, 'need' is sometimes used in an interchangeable way with 'problem' (Compton and Brugha, 1988), to mean 'something demanded' (Bradshaw, 1972), 'want' (Bradshaw, 1972), 'resources offered by professionals' (Armstrong, 1982) and 'a standard defined by a professional' (Bradshaw, 1972). The identification of needs with resources is illustrated well by Brewin *et al.* (1987) who suggested that a need should only be rated as present if there is a standard form of care that would be expected to ameliorate that problem. One wonders whether the patient would agree.

This confused use of the term 'need' stems from the fact that little work had been done on producing a satisfactory theoretical model of need. Waismann (1988) has made an attempt to fill this gap, and has illustrated the complexity of model which is required to describe human need.

The assessment of needs in long-term care has also proved to be difficult because of the lack of a theoretical model. The methods chosen depend in part on the definition of need which has been adopted. For example, if need is thought to be demand, or expressed need, then counting the number of new referrals to a day unit will give one a measure of the need for that unit. In the last few years, two tools have been developed for the assessment of needs of long-term psychiatric patients. Brewin *et al.* (1987) have developed the MRC Needs for Care Assessment, in which staff rate the patient. Waismann and Rowland (1989) have developed a tool that can be used by patients who have difficulty in concentrating when faced with more traditional methods of assessment, which they have used successfully to measure the relative importance that individuals with long-term psychiatric disabilities attribute to various areas of need.

Given the difficulties of defining and measuring need, one might legitimately ask whether it is a useful concept on which to base rehabilitation. One answer to this question lies in a story, for which we are indebted to Dr Len Rowland, that illustrates the difference between a skills and a needs model. A man with long-term psychiatric problems lived on his own in a council flat and visited a Day Care service on a daily basis. The conscientious occupational therapists of the unit assessed his cooking skills and found that he could not cook. So they taught him how to make some meals. Some while later they visited him at home and were distressed to find no food in the house and no evidence of cooking having been done. 'Why don't you make the meals we taught you?' they asked. 'I don't need to,' he said. 'Every evening for years, I've gone along to the local cafe to meet my friends and have something to eat.' He may have lacked the skill of cooking, but his need was to be fed, and this was met nicely by the local cafe, which also provided friendship.

If patients do not acquire or perform skills, then they are often accused of being lazy or 'lacking motivation'. But the real reason may be that the skill is not thought to be important because it does not fulfil a need, or it is thought to be difficult and the need can be met in some easier way.

The concept of need, although poorly understood, is attractive because it forces one to think about the individual, to think beyond specified interventions to creative ways of meeting need and to think in terms of the whole of an individual's life. It also allows one to consider the patient's perspective and his or her quality of life. But a lot more work needs to be done on the definition of need and the development of appropriate measuring devices.

2.2.5 ROLES

A useful but less popular concept for guiding rehabilitation is that of social role. The roles which a person performs provide him/her with a sense of self-worth, particularly if they have little intrinsic belief in his/her own value (Lam and Power, 1991). Rehabilitation is the process of identifying and preventing or minimizing the causes of the severe social disablement which often accompanies psychiatric disorders while at the same time helping the individual to develop or use his/her talents and thus acquire confidence and self-esteem through success in social roles (Wing, 1980). The development and maintenance of social roles is seen as one way of reducing the social disablement brought about by psychiatric illness. One of the greatest difficulties for the person with long-term psychiatric disabilities is to perform roles in a social world (Bennett, 1973).

The roles which we perform determine our status in society. In society roles are arranged in a hierarchy of statuses. An individual may have several roles in different spheres of life: occupational, domestic, social and so on. If we are uanble to meet the expectations of society in our performance of normative roles, then we are regarded as having failed. Within rehabilitation, particular emphasis has been placed on maintaining the occupational role and it is in this sphere that some services, such as the Netherne Rehabilitation Service in East Surrey, have excelled. The primary aim of maintaining the work role has many benefits for somebody with long-term mental health problems, including: aspects of the work itself, such as having to exercise sensory and perceptual judgement; the effect of one's self esteem, which makes it easier to shed the patient role; the protective effect provided by, for example, contacts outside the nuclear family and a social environment with explicit rules (Rowland and Perkins, 1988).

However, Parry (1983) believes that one should not neglect the rehabilitative potential of domestic roles: mother, father, wife, husband. In order to benefit from this potential, systematic analysis of the specific skills and tasks involved in each role is required, along with a description of the structure of the role. Once this has been done the rehabilitative process will involve looking at which elements of the role patients are able to carry out at a particular point in time, which they can learn or develop and which they cannot carry out and so will need support from family or professionals. It is important to remember that the functioning of people with long-term mental health problems fluctuates: there may be times when they can manage most aspects of a particular role, whereas at other times they may need help in some aspects of the role or to have it taken away for a while. When psychotic, a man may be able to maintain his occupational role but not his domestic role, so an appropriate response may be to remove him from home for a while but to support him in continuing to go to work. An implication of the concept of social roles is that one continually assesses the patient's ability to perform each aspect of each role, and increases or decreases the level of support as appropriate.

Within psychiatry, perhaps the most frequently discussed role is the sick role. The argument is that one consequence of thinking of people as mentally **ill** is that we force them into the role of being **sick**, and that there are social expectations of being sick, namely that:

- one is exempt from normal social responsibilities, to a degree appropriate to the nature and severity of the illness;
- one cannot be expected to decide to get better or pull oneself together by an act of will;
- being sick is undesirable, so there is an obligation to want to get well;
- there is an obligation to seek help with getting better from a competent person and to co-operate with the process of getting well (Parsons, 1951).

As a result of its association with psychiatric institutions, mental health workers tend to talk about the taking on of the sick role as something undesirable that is likely to hamper the progress of a patient. On the other hand, we also shake our heads and become annoyed if patients refuse to accept that they are 'ill' and so will not continue to take medication, keep in contact with the psychiatric services or come in to hospital when we think they need to. Perhaps, within rehabilitation, the sick role should be treated like every other potential role for an individual patient. In other words, there must be a constant process of assessment to decide how much, and which aspects, of a particular role an individual should or should not take on. There may be times when it is very important that a person takes on a sick role, but it would be counter to the philosophy of rehabilitation to allow an individual to linger in this role when it is no longer necessary.

The concept of role within rehabilitation can be contrasted with the skills model. The role of mother may be made up of many skills or tasks, but merely carrying out these skills is not enough. 'It is not enough to know how to cook a meal or wash clothes. It is just as important to know when to, or even whether to do that rather than something else, such as spending an hour playing with a toddler or baby.' (Parry, 1983)

2.3 GUIDING PHILOSOPHIES

2.3.1 DEINSTITUTIONALIZATION

Deinstitutionalization is the contraction of traditional institutional settings, with the concurrent expansion of community-based services (Bachrach, 1976). It has been the most important influence upon the changes which have taken place in mental health policy and practice in recent years. Bachrach (1988) has argued that there are three identifiable ways of looking at deinstitutionalization – as a fact, as a process and as a philosophy – and each of these will be examined in turn.

(a) Fact

Deinstitutionalization is a fact, as shown by an objective series of events which have taken place, and which continue to take place. In Britain, as in other countries, there has been a continuous decline in the number of psychiatric hospital beds available in psychiatry. The British government, in the White Paper *Better Services for the Mentally Ill* (Department of Health and Social Security, 1975), established a target of 47 900 inpatient psychiatric beds after the completion of the current programme of hospital closure. To date, approximately 84% of the planned reduction from the high point of 148 000 in 1954 has taken place, and only the final sixth of long-stay patients remains to be located (Thornicroft and Bebbington, 1989). In the USA, of an estimated 1 700 000–2 400 000 people with chronic illness only 116 000 remained in state mental hospitals by 1983 (Bachrach, 1986a). In 1955 23% of the USA's services were outpatient, and in 1988 80% (Bachrach, 1988). In Italy, as a result of hospital closure since 1978, there has been a progressive decline in the number of public mental hospital beds, to a level of 0.76 per thousand of the population by 1983 (Tansella *et al.*, 1987). These three countries are not the exception – deinstitutionalization is an international fact.

(b) Process

Deinstitutionalization is a process of social change, from one orientation in patient care to another, namely from care based on psychiatric institutions to 'care in the community'. As stated above, the process of deinstitutionalization is not just about reducing beds, but also about the setting up of alternative services. Thus it affects the lives not only of those individuals who have to move out of hospital but also those individuals who have never lived in a psychiatric asylum and whose lives will be shaped by the new forms of service provision. In Britain, as in other countries, the process has been pushed and moulded by Government policy. Jones (1988) described the process of change which was envisaged and which is embodied in Government documents. What can be seen is that from at least as early as the publication of *A Hospital Plan* (Ministry of Health, 1962) and *Health and Welfare: the Development of Community Care* (Ministry of Health, 1963) it has been envisaged that hospital services should be restricted largely to the acute sector, based in District General Hospitals, with the transfer of chronic patients to local authority care. This conceptualization was made law in the National Health Service and Community Care Act (Department of Health, 1990).

It would be reasonable to assume that evaluation of the effects of this major change would be built in to the international process of deinstitutionalization, with the results altering or, if appropriate, stopping or delaying the process. However, despite the existence of some major studies of the process and its effects, such as the Worcester Development Project (Milner, 1991) and the TAPS Project in North London (Beecham *et al.*, 1990), the deinstitutionalization movement, once started, has gained its own momentum (Bachrach, 1988) and the findings of such studies have had, and are having, little effect on the process.

(c) Philosophy

Deinstitutionalization is a philosophy which has its roots in the anti-psychiatry movement of the 1950s and 1960s. The mentally ill were seen as victims who would receive more humane care if the large psychiatric asylums no longer existed. Deinstitutionalization was not, and is not, a response to any research findings that living in institutions is bad for people with long-term and severe mental health problems. Instead, Thornicroft and Bebbington (1989) argued that deinstitutionalization began because it was seen as the only humane response to the severe overcrowding that existed in the psychiatric asylums and that, thereafter, the following influences came into play.

Sociological arguments.   Criticism of the negative effects of prolonged stays in institutions emerged; for example, Barton (1959) described what he called 'institutional neurosis', a 'disease' caused by psychiatric institutions, with symptoms of apathy, lack of initiative and loss of interest. Goffman (1961) developed the concept of the 'total institution', a central element of which was that people were shaped into the role of psychiatric patient by aspects of the institution such as being treated *en bloc* rather than having individual needs met.

Financial considerations.   It was assumed that care in the community would be cheaper than care in large asylums, particularly because, in Britain, most of the asylums which had been built around the turn of the century were in drastic need of repair. Studies continue to be carried out to investigate the financial implications of the new service provision (e.g. Beecham *et al.*, 1990).

Treatment development.   Several developments in treatment made deinstitutionalization seem more possible. After the development of chlorpromazine in 1952, its use rapidly became widespread (Jones, 1972). There were also developments in patient management, with the introduction of industrial therapy, behaviour therapy, therapeutic communities and so on.

Legal influences.   The 1959 Mental Health Act embodied an assumption (which was made explicit in the 1975 amendment to the act) that community mental health care is the most effective and humane form of care for most mentally ill people.

Hospital enquiries.   There was a series of enquiries into malpractice in British hospitals for the mentally ill. Martin (1984) has documented 14 investigations and enquiries in Britain between 1969 and 1980. He found some recurring themes associated with established cases of ill-treatment: isolation of the institutions, lack of staff support, poor reporting procedures, a failure of leadership, ineffectual administration, inadequate financial resources, the divided loyalties of trade unions, poor staff training and negligent individuals (Thornicroft and Bebbington, 1989). The effect of such enquiries was to reinforce the developing view that the large institutions were harmful.

Deinstitutionalization, therefore, had humane goals, and it began with hope and optimism. It was based on many assumptions, rather than on research findings. Whatever the results of evaluation, the process is speeding along with increasing momentum and it is unlikely to be reversible.

2.3.2 COMMUNITY CARE

Rehabilitation is not the same as community care. This may sound like stating the obvious, but as we have already seen, rehabilitation is often wrongly thought to mean resettlement outside hospital 'in the community', and from this point its confusion with community care is easy. If community care is not rehabilitation, what is it? One answer to the question is that community care is the law, both in Britain and in many other countries. In Britain, the National Health Service and Community Care Act (Department of Health, 1990) laid down not only a new structure for the organization of care for those people who had in the past been cared for on long-stay hospital wards: the long-term mentally ill, people with learning disabilities and the elderly. The emphasis is on care outside hospital as far as possible, provided locally, and with a shift of responsibility from the Health Service to Social Services. So here community care seems to mean 'not in hospital', and 'not health service', although it is never defined explicitly in the Act.

To say that Community Care is the law is not, of course, an adequate answer. Rowland et al. (1992) have provided a helpful unpacking of the uses to which the term is put:

Non-hospital care.   At times, such as in the 1990 NHS and Community Care Act, 'community care' means little more than 'not hospital care'. The danger here is that the 'care' bit is forgotten. A good example of this might be the increase in the incidence of mental illness found amongst the homeless, both in Britain and in the USA (Bachrach, 1984; Abdul-Hamid and McCarthy, 1989; Bates and Walsh, 1989).

Care by the community.   Particularly in the early days, 'community care' was idealistically assumed to mean 'care by the community'. This is, however, rarely the case. The elements of community care are most often set up by, and receive continual support from, hospitals and hospital staff (Rowland et al., 1992). Although some patients return to or remain living with their relatives, the majority do not (Conning and Rowland, 1992). Perhaps the best example of care by the community is to be found in Geel in Belgium (Rowland, Zeelan and Waismann, 1992). Here, since the thirteenth century, long-stay patients from all over Belgium have been placed with foster families supported by a nurse who visits on a regular basis. Although hospital beds are available if the need arises, the majority of people who are admitted return to their foster families. The 'care by the community' appears to be successfully keeping people out of hospital.

Care in communities.   A frequent response to community care is the idea that people should be cared for 'in communities' such as group homes, hostels, day centres or 'therapeutic communities'. However, taking group living arrangements as an example, the 'community' aspect may have less benefits than we assume. Most residents do not consider themselves to have close friendships with other residents (Pritlove, 1983; Hill, 1988), although they may go out together sometimes and help each other with practical problems (Pritlove, 1983). Some individuals cannot cope with the socially stimulating environment created by group living (Falloon and Marshall, 1983) and many people who live in hostels or group homes would prefer to live alone (Lehman, Ward and Linn, 1982; Kay and Legg, 1986).

It is frequently assumed that community care will guarantee successful care. This, however, depends on the way it is set up. Community care can be applied to any client group; here we are concerned with people with long-term and severe mental health problems. Bachrach (1980, 1989, 1991) has suggested 13 principles upon which to base service provision for this client group.

- Assign top priority to the care of the most severely impaired: target those who are chronically and persistently ill.
- Link realistically to other resources in the community.
- Either by itself or in combination with other resources to which it is linked, the service should attempt to provide for its patients the full range of functions that are associated with institutional care, namely: long-term care; asylum or a place of refuge; accommodation and food; medical treatment; social and vocational help; supervised accommodation (custody) for those who have broken the law or engage in behaviour which will not be tolerated elsewhere; a comprehensive service; and secure employment for professionals.

- Provide personally tailored treatment regimes, whether chemotherapy, psychotherapy, psychosocial rehabilitation and/or some combination of these and other treatment modalities.
- Tailor the service to the local realities of the community in which the service is located.
- Employ trained staff who are attuned to the unique survival problems of chronic mental patients living in non-institutional settings. Provide them with special training which includes strategies for dealing not only with problems in patient care but also with staff issues, like burn-out, that affect their performance.
- The service should be tied to a complement of hospital beds.
- Have an ongoing internal assessment mechanism that permits continuous self-monitoring.
- Emphasize chronic mental patients' strengths.
- Employ assertive outreach.
- Employ aggressive leadership in caring for the chronic mentally ill.
- The service should be eclectic and receptive to various kinds of assistance.
- Cultivate the ability to think ahead seriously, objectively and without bias about future treatment needs.

2.3.3 NORMALIZATION

Normalization or, as it has been referred to more recently, 'social role valorization' (Wolfensberger, 1983) is not a model but a guiding principle. The idea was developed by Wolfensberger (1970), who defined it as 'utilization of means which are as culturally normative as possible, in order to establish, enable, or support behaviours, appearances and interpretations which are as culturally normative as possible', or more simply 'the use of culturally valued means in order to enable people to live culturally valued lives (Wolfensberger, 1980).

However, by Wolfensberger's own admission, the choice of the word 'normalization' was an unfortunate one, because it is derived from the word 'normal' and so has been taken to mean making people normal, or fitting a person to the statistical norm of the society. He pointed out that this is a naive and invalid interpretation of the principle, particularly because what society expects of someone, and values, is quite often not the same as the statistical norm.

The principle of normalization can be applied to any individual or group of individuals who are devalued, although its central concern was with the right of mentally disabled people to live full lives. It sees the social value that is given by society to the experience of long-term mental illness as the key to understanding much of the difficulty faced by disabled individuals. The goal is the enhancement in value of the social role assigned to people who use mental health services, who are at risk of social devaluation (Pilling, 1991).

In many respects some of the ideas based upon normalization have become part of day-to-day practice, without reference to the principle itself. For example, housing associations do not put up large signs outside their hostels announcing their presence in an ordinary street. Perhaps this is one of the principle's strengths – it has become part of everyday thinking. Its other advantages are that: it demands that patients are thought about as people; it concentrates on people's strengths; it reduces stigma and encourages integration with society; it can be used in conjunction with any of the therapeutic models which have been discussed above.

However, in practice, the principle is often applied in a naive way, in which case it has several disadvantages. For example, it has been used to support an argument that if people with long-term psychiatric disabilities are put in 'normal' settings (that is, not in hospital), they will become 'normal', and so it can be used as an excuse for not providing adequate long-term services, including inpatient beds when necessary. It is also possible to ignore the fact that long-term psychiatric patients have problems and disabilities that need to be treated. For example, a hospital sheltered workshop for the most disabled clients was to move on to an industrial estate; the staff were debating whether or not depot medication should be given in the workshop to the few patients who needed it. Apparently applying the principle of normalization, some staff said that it was inappropriate for the injections to be given in a workshop, so the patients should go to the depot clinic at a day unit two miles away. However, it was pointed out that these patients were unreliable with appointments and had difficulty with public transport, and so would be unlikely to turn up regularly at a clinic for their injections. Here the choice was between not giving injections in a workshop, with the consequence of making it unlikely that the patients would receive the medication they needed, or having a visiting nurse discreetly slip into the rest room to give the injections. Perhaps the real choice is between whether being well and being able to hold down one's job is more socially valued than not giving injections in a work setting. Meeting the needs of the patient must come first, although one will want to meet these needs in as socially valued a way as possible.

REFERENCES

Abdul-Hamid W. and McCarthy, M. (1989) Community psychiatric care for homeless people in inner London. *Health Trends*, **21**, 67–69.

Anthony, W.A. (1977) Psychological rehabilitation: a concept in need of a method. *American Psychologist*, **Aug**, 658–662.

Anthony, W.A., Cohen, M.R. and Cohen, B.F. (1984) Psychiatric rehabilitation, in *The Chronic Mental Patient: Five Years Later*, (ed. J.A. Talbott), Grune & Stratton, Orlando, FL, ch. 10.

Anthony, W.A. and Liberman, R.P. (1986) The practice of psychiatric rehabilitation: historical conceptual and research base. *Schizophrenia Bulletin*, **12**(4), 542–559.

Anthony, W.A. and Margules, A. (1974) Toward improving the efficacy of psychiatric rehabilitation: a skills training approach. *Rehabilitation Psychology*, **21**, 101–105.

Armstrong, P.F. (1982) The myth of meeting needs in adult education and community development. *Critical Social Policy*, **2**(2), 24–27.

Bachrach, L. (1976) *Deinstitutionalization: an analytical review and sociological perspective*, US Department of Health, Education and Welfare, NIMH, Rockville, MD.

Bachrach, L. (1980) Overview: model programmes for chronic mental patients. *American Journal of Psychiatry*, **137**(9), 1023–1031.

Bachrach, L. (1984) Interpreting research on the homeless mentally ill: some caveats. *Hospital and Community Psychiatry*, **35**, 914–917.

Bachrach, L. (1986a) The future of the state mental hospital. *Hospital and Community Psychiatry*, **37**, 467–474.

Bachrach, L. (1986b) Dimensions of disability in the chronic mentally ill. *Hospital and Community Psychiatry*, **37**(10), 981–982.

Bachrach, L. (1988) *Aspects of Deinstitutionalization*. Paper given at the Institute of Psychiatry, University of London, 9.11.88.

Bachrach, L. (1989) The legacy of model programs. *Hospital and Community Psychiatry*, **40**(3), 234–235.

Bachrach, L. (1991) The 13th principle. *Hospital and Community Psychiatry*, **42**(12), 1205–1206.

Barton, R. (1959) *Institutional Neurosis*, John Wright, Bristol.

Bates, P. and Walsh, M. (1989) *Empty Premises – Empty Promises*, Benefits Research Unit Occasional Paper, 1/89, Nottingham.

Beecham, J., Anderson, J., Dayson, D. *et al.* (1990) The TAPS Project, III. Predicting the community costs of closing psychiatric hospitals. *British Journal of Psychiatry*, **157**, 661–670.

Bennett, D.H. (1973) Rehabilitation in psychiatry. *Occupational Therapy*, **April**, 290–291.

Bennett, D.H. (1978) Social forms of psychiatric treatment, in *Schizophrenia: Towards a New Synthesis*, (ed. J.K. Wing), Academic Press, London.

Bennett, D.H. (1983) The historical development of rehabilitation services, in *Theory and Practice of Psychiatric Rehabilitation*, (eds F.N. Watts and D.H. Bennett), John Wiley & Sons, Chichester.

Bradshaw, J. (1972) The concept of social need. *New Society*, **30**, 640–643.

Brewin, C.R., Wing, J.K., Mangen, S.P. *et al.* (1987) Principles and practices of measuring needs of the long-term mentally ill: the MRC needs for care assessment. *Psychological Medicine*, **17**, 971–981.

Compton, S. and Brugha, T. (1988) Problems in monitoring needs for care of long-term psychiatric patients: evaluating a service for casual attenders. *Social Psychiatry and Psychiatric Epidemiology*, **23**, 121–125.

Conning, A.M. and Rowland, L.A. (1992) Staff attitudes and the provision of individualised care: what determines what we do for people with long-term psychiatric disabilities? *Journal of Mental Health*, **1**, 71–80.

Department of Health (1990) *National Health Service and Community Care Act 1990*, HMSO, London.

Department of Health (1991) *The Patient's Charter*, HMSO, London.

Department of Health and Social Security (1975) *Better Services for the Mentally Ill*, Cmnd 6233, HMSO, London.

Falloon, I.R. and Marshall, G.N. (1983) Residential care and social behaviour: a study of rehabilitation needs. *Psychological Medicine*, **13**, 341–347.

Farkas, M. (1990) La rehabilitación del paciente mental cronico en la comunidad, Junta de Andalucía. Unpublished conference paper, Universidad Internacional Mendez Pelayo, Seville.

Goffman, I. (1961) *Asylums: Essays on the Social Situation of Mental Patients and Other Inmates*. Penguin Books, Harmondsworth, Middlesex.

Hill, B.A. (1988) Factors influencing satisfaction and successful placement in hostels for people with a long-term psychiatric disability. University of London. MSc thesis.

Jones, K. (1972) *A History of the Mental Health Service*, Routledge and Kegan Paul, London.

Jones, K. (1988) *Experience in Mental Health: Community Care and Social Policy*, Sage Publications, London, Ch. 2.

Kay, A. and Legg, C. (1986) *Discharged to the Community: A Review of Housing and Support in London for People Leaving Psychiatric Care*, Good Practices in Mental Health, London.

Khwaja, A. (1985) Communication between staff and patients in a setting designed to promote normal behaviour. University of London. MPhil thesis.

Lam, D.H. and Power, M.J. (1991) A questionnaire designed to assess roles and goals: a preliminary study. *British Journal of Medical Psychology*, **64**, 359–373.

Lehman, A.F., Ward, N.C. and Linn, L.S. (1982) Chronic mental patients: the quality of life issue. *American Journal of Psychiatry*, **139**, 1271–1276.

Liberman, R.P., Falloon, I.R.H. and Wallace, C.J. (1984) Drug-psychosocial interventions in the treatment of schizophrenia, in *The Chronically Mentally Ill: Research and Services*, (ed. M. Mirabi), SP Medical and Scientific Books, New York.

Liberman, R.P., Mueser, K.T., Wallace, C.J. *et al.* (1986) Training skills in the psychiatrically disabled: learning, coping and competence. *Schizophrenia Bulletin*, **12**(4), 631–647.

Martin, L. (1984) *Hospitals in Trouble*, Blackwell, Oxford.

Milner, G. (1991) The Worcester Development Project 20 years on, in *The Closure of Mental Hospitals*, (eds P. Hall and I.F. Brockington), Gaskell, London.

Ministry of Health (1962) A Hospital Plan for England and Wales, Cmnd 1604, HMSO, London.

Ministry of Health (1963) Health and Welfare: the Development of Community Care, Cmnd 1973, HMSO, London.

Parry, G. (1983) Domestic roles, in *Theory and Practice of Psychiatric Rehabilitation*, (eds F.N. Watts and D.H. Bennett), John Wiley & Sons, Chichester.

Parsons, T. (1951) *The Social System*, Routledge and Kegan Paul, London.

Pilling, S. (1991) *Rehabilitation and Community Care*, Routledge, London.

Pritlove, J. (1983) Accommodation without resident staff for ex-psychiatric patients. *British Journal of Social Work*, **13**, 75–92.

Rowland, L. and Perkins, R. (1988) You can't eat, drink or make love eight hours a day: the value of work in psychiatry. *Health Trends*, **20**, 75–80.

Rowland, L.A., Zeelan, J. and Waismann, L.C. (1992) Patterns of service for the long-term mentally ill in Europe. *British Journal of Clinical Psychiatry*, **31**, 405–417.

Summers, F. and Hersh, S. (1983) Psychiatric chronicity and diagnosis. *Schizophrenia Bulletin*, **9**, 123–133.

Tansella, M., De Salvia, D. and Williams, P. (1987) The Italian psychiatric reform: some quantitative evidence. *Social Psychiatry*, **22**, 37–48.

Thapa, K. and Rowland, L.A. (1989) Quality of life perspectives in long-term care: staff and patient perceptions. *Acta Psychiatrica Scandinavica*, **80**, 267–271.

Thornicroft, G. and Bebbington, P. (1989) Deinstitutionalisation – from hospital closure to service development. *British Journal of Psychiatry*, **155**, 739–753.

Waismann, L.C. (1988) Needs and other motivational processes in long-term psychiatric patients in an era of community care. University of London. PhD thesis.

Waismann, L.C. and Rowland, L.A. (1989) Ranking of needs: a new method of assessment for use with chronic psychiatric patients. *Acta Psychiatrica Scandinavica*, **80**, 260–266.

Wing, J.K. (1978) Clinical concepts of schizophrenia, in *Schizophrenia: Towards a New Synthesis* (ed. J.K. Wing), Academic Press, London.

Wing, J.K. (1980) *Psychiatric Rehabilitation in the 1980s. Report of the Working Party on Rehabilitation*, Royal College of Psychiatrists, London.

Wing, J.K. (1981) Recent advances in understanding schizophrenia, in *Rehabilitation of Patients with Schizophrenia and Depression*, (eds J.K. Wing, P. Kielohlz and W.M. Zinn), Hans Stubler, Bern.

Wolfensberger, W. (1970) The principle of normalization and its implications to psychiatric services. *American Journal of Psychiatry*, **127**, 291–297.

Wolfensberger, W. (1980) The definition of normalization: update, problems, disagreements and misunderstandings, in *Normalization, Social Integration and Community Services* (eds R.J. Flynn and K.E. Nitsch), University Park Press, Baltimore, MD.

Wolfensberger, W. (1983) Social role valorization: a proposed new term for the principle of normalization. *Mental Retardation*, **21**, 234–239.

Wood, P.H.N. and Badley, E.M. (1978) An epidemiological appraisal of disablement, in *Recent Advances in Community Medicine*, (ed. H.E. Bennett), Churchill Livingstone, Edinburgh.

Rehabilitation assessment

3

Assessment is the backbone of rehabilitation practice; no rehabilitation programme is viable without an integral system of assessment. It is the essential first step in the diagnostic process, the basis for prescribing interventions, for monitoring results and for predicting outcome. Since social disablement presents a highly complex picture of interwoven clinical impairments and secondary disabilities, aggregate assessments of its constituents have to be made; these include appraisals of the disabled person's psychiatric and physical state, his/her current and premorbid social functioning, attitudes to his/her disabilities and response to help, as well as his/her social environment. A comprehensive view of all these facets of disablement can only be made with any degree of accuracy by the pooled contributions of people involved in the rehabilitation process, each of whom must have a working knowledge of assessment methods.

In an excellent introductory account, Hall (1981) outlined the purposes of rehabilitation assessments, which include judging the individual's level of disability, planning a rehabilitation programme and observing progress over time, as well as the planning of services and conducting research; it also discusses the targets of assessment techniques. This chapter will consider these aspects and their implications in some detail.

3.1 THE PROCESS OF ASSESSMENT

3.1.1 THE AIMS OF REHABILITATION ASSESSMENT

People with psychiatric disabilities are referred to rehabilitation services for a variety of reasons; they may be referred specifically for skills training in the spheres of personal care, domestic and occupational tasks, money management, leisure time, work activities and management of long-term medication; some are referred as a last resort, because of their intractable difficult or 'challenging' behaviour. Other reasons may be vaguely expressed and concepts such as 'stabilization', 'improving social functioning' or 'independence' may appear on referral forms. A sizable proportion of referrals are expressly made for placement in suitable accommodation or occupational settings (Ekdawi, 1990). There may be other, covert, reasons for the referral, for example releasing a bed in a busy acute admissions ward. An understanding of the purpose of the referral may guide the assessors in the emphasis they place on the areas to be assessed.

There are several interconnected reasons for making an individual rehabilitation assessment.

1. It is important **to reach a diagnosis of the main problems** so that the dimensions of the social disablement are mapped out, which makes it possible

2. **to determine the most appropriate interventions** with the best chance of improving function for the present time and those which may potentially be needed in future, as well as areas where interventions may not be useful or necessary. An inventory of such interventions would include those directed at the individual's environment, such as family work, sheltered employment or sheltered residential accommodation.

3. **A tentative prognostic statement can then be made** regarding the probability of the success of these interventions, on the long-term outcome and on the need for further interventions in terms of treatment and management. It is as well to remember, however, that predicting results and outcome is exceedingly difficult and that longer-term predictions have a greater margin of error.

4. Individual assessments are the basis for **action directed at organization and service change**. Accumulated information that highlights the needs of a group of disabled individuals may lead to changes in the planned direction of a service's provisions – for instance, expanding the number of social clubs or employing more technical staff in a sheltered workshop.

5. Assessments are also **essential for research** since the rationale for the development of more precise assessment methods or for developing more effective interventions has to be constantly informed by research evidence; the assessment of groups of patients in three hospitals, for example, has shown the importance of constructive occupation in reducing disability (Wing and Brown, 1970), and the assessment of community patients has emphasized the positive effects of family interventions in reducing relapse rates (Falloon, 1990). Both these examples, in turn, have had wide-ranging effects on rehabilitation interventions and services.

3.1.2 BACKGROUND INFORMATION FOR REHABILITATION ASSESSMENT

Assessment is the process of balancing several variables which leads to an informed judgement. In a rehabilitation assessment, this involves the conceptualization of factors which contribute to the disabled person's difficulties in social functioning; underlying this judgement is an implication that the service may offer suitable interventions to enable him/her to improve his/her performance within appropriate environments, so that these difficulties may be reduced or eliminated. The first step towards making this judgement is to gather essential information from reliable sources on the person's past history, the current level of social functioning, the social circumstances and the state of physical and mental health. It is also important to include information on the person's own views, attitudes and wishes for the future. The process of information gathering will therefore comprise a number of core elements.

- A history should be taken of the individual's psychiatric disorder and past physical illness, and the family and social background prior to the presumed onset of illness. This includes: any family history of psychiatric disorder and family relationships and contacts; educational attainments and employment history; interpersonal relationships and adequacy of past performance within social roles. Relevant chronological details of the individual's past treatment and contact with psychiatric services including hospital admission are documented, together with reported factors which may have had a bearing on the course of the illness and the frequency of contact with services.
- Current social functioning and environmental factors that may have affected the performance of social roles should be established. Particular attention is paid to the duration and stability of personal relationships and employment since they have prognostic implications.
- The psychiatric diagnosis and current symptoms should be noted and, more importantly, the degree to which these may influence behaviour; this is of particular relevance because behaviour rather than symptoms by themselves is a decisive factor in community survival and job tenure.
- Information should be sought which might help in estimating the person's insight into his/her difficulties, reactions to his/her disabilities, and levels of confidence and self-esteem; this type of information is far from easy to elicit, but a guess can be made, based on the person's past attempts to form relationships, to seek employment or to exploit sources of help.

All these elements are inter-related; the difficulty in gathering accurate information about each aspect is compounded by many factors, not least of which is the variable reliability of the sources of information. Case records of long-term patients, for instance, are notorious for the paucity of information relevant to rehabilitation. An unobtrusive patient with many years' hospital stay may only accrue a slim volume of scanty notes; the weighty hospital records of another patient may be rich in their descriptions of symptoms, incidents and physical complaints and sparse on even simple, straightforward demographic details. Essential facts of the past history may be missing and the chronology of life events may be muddled; it is also sometimes extraordinarily difficult to elicit accurate information, for example, on periods of unemployment or on the reasons for prescribing or changing the dosage of medication and the effects of such changes. It is also well-known that obtaining information covering long periods of time from the person concerned or from other informants can be highly problematic, particularly in the 'softer' areas of personal relationships, which are often coloured by subjective opinion; moreover, different informants may give conflicting accounts since behaviour fluctuates over time and varies in different situations. While it is important, in history-taking, to enquire about environmental factors which place demands on the individual or which may be supportive or, alternatively, noxious, care must be taken in teasing out and excluding facile speculation; a description of the actions of a concerned mother, for instance, is preferable to calling her overprotective.

In conclusion, the recording of historical data for assessments should be as clear and as objective as possible so that it forms a rational basis of information for assessment by other methods.

3.1.3 ASSESSMENT METHODS – GENERAL PRINCIPLES

Rehabilitation assessments rely on accurate observation and on the use of sound, practical interview and rating procedures. The various aspects of social disablement make it necessary for assessments to be carried out by a variety of personnel; these are normally medical and nursing staff, clinical psychologists, occupational therapists and social workers as well as informal carers and, whenever possible, the disabled person. If appropriate, additional assessments are made by physiotherapists, speech therapists, teachers and voluntary workers. The assessments are collated so that the specifications of the person's strengths and weaknesses are delineated. Some of the assessment methods used in various contexts will be described in more detail later; however, common underlying principles and concerns will now be discussed.

A variety of assessment procedures are practised within rehabilitation services; these mainly consist of the use of interviews (structured, semi-structured or unstructured) and of rating scales. In a review of over 200 articles concerned with assessment procedures used in studies of long-term patients, Hall (1976) made several valuable recommendations on the application of assessment rating scales.

- More than one type of assessment method should be used.
- Only standardized assessment methods should be used; any modifications of these methods should only be made on the basis of careful rationale and they should be published.
- Measures should be valid and reliable and they should be sensitive to change.

It should also be noted that, for the purpose of clinical practice as distinct from research, the methods used should be easy to administer and economical on time and they should require neither elaborate equipment nor extensive training of the assessors. In addition, research and clinical experience have shown that, in using any assessment procedure, the following points should also be considered.

- In rehabilitation practice, snapshot assessments are of only limited use. Ideally, an assessment procedure should have some retrospective and some prospective elements; this means that it covers a specified period of observation and that it takes into account potential future fluctuations and change. Clearly, the observation time has to be relevant to the focus of assessment; a month's record of attendance at work may be long enough as an indicator of punctuality, while the same period may be too brief to gauge the effects of an intervention used to manage infrequent aggressive episodes. To be meaningful, most assessments have to be repeated at intervals; however, the intervals should not be too short, since changes are, more often than not, very slow.
- It is often pointed out that assessments concentrate, in the main, on deficits and abnormalities while neglecting, or only paying lip service to, assets and strengths. This is particularly evident in some of the methods of assessing social performance. Assessors may underestimate a person's level of competence to perform certain role tasks because of the lack of opportunity to practise them, so that, for example, astonishment may be expressed on learning that a patient was able to cope remarkably well alone at home while his parents were on holiday. Conversely, competence levels may be misjudged; a good level of work competence in a hospital workshop, for example, may not guarantee similar performance in a community sheltered workshop. Whenever

possible, therefore, assessments should be carried out in different, realistic, settings.

- Poor task performance may not only be caused by lack of skills or disuse atrophy of skills; it is sometimes due to lack of interest, poor motivation or personal low priority. Much staff effort, for example, can be wasted in training a man to cook if he intends to live in lodgings where meals are provided or if he strongly believes that cooking is a woman's job (Chapter 2).
- Assessors have to be alert to the fact that assessments are not simply inventories of behaviours, but imply whole judgements based on certain expectations; low levels of social performance, for example, that may be tolerated in some cultural settings or within certain families, may be quite unacceptable in others.
- There is a risk that assessments may become just another ritual of routine work; the purpose of the assessment should always be kept in mind and the conclusions drawn from it should be clearly and accurately recorded in the context of the rehabilitation plan. Furthermore, the assessments skills of an assessor may decline with the passage of time if they are not monitored – familiarity could breed perfunctoriness.

3.1.4 THE INITIAL ASSESSMENT

People referred to rehabilitation services are usually assessed, initially, at a screening interview prior to their transfer to the care of the rehabilitation team. This screening interview can take various forms depending on the type of care or facility for which they are considered, and it is usually preceded by a written request, or a referral form, from the referring agent. This should include basic data about the person's name, age, address, marital status and agencies currently involved in care, together with a brief summary of the person's clinical state, treatment, including medication, home circumstances and current work and leisure activities. The main aims of the referral should be stated.

It is desirable that referrals should be received at a central point, such as a ward or a day hospital, by a small multidisciplinary assessment team representing the rehabilitation team as a whole. The assessment team may then arrange for the referred person to pay an informal visit to the facility which will be the main base for his rehabilitation programme; the visit may include attending a community meeting or joining in a communal meal, and the person may be given written information on the range of choices that could be offered by the service. A more formal assessment interview should be arranged by the assessment team to meet the referred person, preferably accompanied by someone who knows him or her; the purpose of this initial interview is to exchange information and answer questions arising from the referral and to briefly explore the person's main difficulties, needs and wishes. At the conclusion of the interview, the participants jointly reach a decision regarding the appropriate course of action, which may be a recommendation for transfer to the care of the rehabilitation service or, alternatively, for the referring team to implement certain changes in the current care programme, possibly with a view to reassessment at a future date. The decision should be relayed to the referring agent in writing. Occasionally, a trial period in a chosen rehabilitation facility is agreed before care is formally accepted by the rehabilitation team. This is followed by more formalized assessment procedures over a defined period of time, in preparation for discussion at a multidisciplinary rehabilitation assessment conference.

3.1.5 THE ASSESSMENT CONFERENCE – AN EXAMPLE

When a date for the multidisciplinary assessment conference is decided, the person, relatives, if appropriate, and members of the team are notified in advance. It should be clearly understood by all concerned that the conference's main objectives are to identify the person's disabilities and strengths, based on the assessments, to set agreed rehabilitation goals and to choose interventions which may achieve the goals. Documented relevant information is prepared by members of the team for presentation at the conference; it is suggested that this should include:

- medical and psychiatric history, current clinical state and current treatment;
- social and family circumstances gleaned from social reports and family interviews;
- educational attainments, work history (including number and duration of jobs, preferred jobs and periods of unemployment) and current work performance;
- levels of social performance as assessed by observation and rating scales;
- any other observations that may assist in the identification of the individual's needs;
- the person's own views on his/her needs, priorities and future aspirations.

(a) Suggested check list

Before the presentation, documented assessments embracing three essential aspects of the case are prepared:

- present mental state (for example, Krawiecka rating), current medication and its side-effects if any, and current physical health;
- social assessment, including family circumstances, levels of social functioning and symptomatic behaviour, financial resources and current social networks (for example, Morningside Rehabilitation Status Scales);
- work assessment, including current work performance and vocational assessment.

As in any other aspects of the rehabilitation programme, the assessed person should be encouraged to participate in preparing for the conference; the person is more likely to become involved if consulted and if offered the opportunity to make choices and less likely to experience feelings of anxiety and frustration if his/her views are fully considered.

Whenever possible, the assessed person should take an active part in discussing proposed interventions with the team at the conference.

During the conference, discussions should focus on the person's main rehabilitation needs; this may be facilitated by means of a check list of interventions which may be considered, such as:

- additional specific assessment;
- symptom relief and management of self-medication;
- choice of suitable accommodation;
- work placements;
- education and training courses;
- help with long-term relationships;
- assistance with state benefits and money management;
- introduction to other agencies concerned with psychiatric disability;
- maintenance of continuity of treatment, care and support;
- involvement of the family in the rehabilitation process.

A suggested rehabilitation plan is then formulated consisting of specified aims and defined steps to achieve them. The plan should be clearly recorded in a way which can be readily understood by all involved; descriptions of the aims and interventions should be brief, realistic and unambiguous; vague goals such as 'to improve self-care' or 'to increase confidence' should be avoided. The number of proposed interventions should not exceed four or five items: a long list can be confusing and easily forgotten. A copy of the agreed plan is given to the person and to the members of the team who have a responsibility in its implementation.

A summary of the content of the conference is written, preferably on one sheet of paper, under clear headings (history, social circumstances, global ratings, rehabilitation plan, etc.) and it should include a date for the next conference when modifications in the plan might be considered in the light of further assessments.

3.1.6 REVIEWS

Multidisciplinary review meetings are often a regular feature of rehabilitation services' timetables. They are usually in the form of 'ward rounds' where a number of disabled people are briefly discussed, and their main function is to monitor and to respond to changes. It is essential, at each review, to mention each individual on the case list so that the unobtrusive person who is 'no trouble' is not forgotten.

A calendar of such reviews would involve groups of users of a particular element of the service such as a hostel, a hospital ward or a day care facility; the frequency of the reviews is determined by the needs of each group. It is inevitable that overlaps will occur – for example, the same person may be reviewed twice, once as a hostel resident and again as a sheltered workshop worker, but there are advantages in monitoring social performance in different settings and there is less likelihood of some people slipping through the net. A documented summary of each review should be made available to those team members who are particularly involved with the persons reviewed.

3.2 ASSESSMENT METHODS

3.2.1 SCHEDULES AND RATING SCALES

(a) Psychiatric assessment

The type and degree of severity of psychiatric symptoms may significantly affect the disabled person's social behaviour and response to rehabilitation interventions. The symptomatic behaviour displayed by grossly deluded or profoundly depressed persons may make it difficult for them to function at a reasonable level or to benefit from rehabilitation measures such as skills training; in fact these interventions may exacerbate positive symptoms and increase the severity of maladaptive behaviour, and without adequate treatment directed at symptom relief or symptom control a rehabilitation programme may be ineffective or positively harmful.

On the other hand, negative symptoms of schizophrenia have been shown to become more marked in the presence of low levels of social stimulation; in addition, prolonged attempts at energetic medical treatment of these symptoms is often counterproductive and may increase dependency. The assessment of the mental state of people with chronic psychiatric disorder, therefore, has to be thorough and it should take into account the type of current symptoms, their severity and their likely impact on behaviour; it should also include an evaluation of the likely effects of long-term treatment. Assessments should be repeated at intervals over a long period of time by professionals who have some knowledge of the patient, since changes in the clinical picture may be slow and subtle, and in view of the fact that many psychiatrically disabled people find it difficult to communicate their distress – the gap between 'felt' need and 'expressed' need (Bradshaw, 1972) may mean that important changes could escape notice. This is particularly relevant, for instance, in the detection of depressive symptoms in people disabled by chronic schizophrenic illness; it should be remembered that depression contributes to increased morbidity levels and high suicide rates in this group. Another example is the occasionally overlooked cognitive impairment which may exist concurrently with symptoms of schizophrenia and which may adversely affect response to rehabilitation interventions.

The psychiatric assessment should include a comment on the individual's degree of insight, as this may greatly influence his/her response to the rehabilitation plans.

The difficulties inherent in the clinical assessment of people disabled by psychiatric illness by means of the traditional mental state examination have led to the use of more sophisticated methods and assessment schedules specifically developed for this purpose. Some examples will now be considered.

- The Present State Examination (PSE) developed in the 1960s (Kendall, Everitt and Cooper, 1968) is a detailed, comprehensive instrument which requires training. It is an example of a good assessment procedure mainly used for research purposes.
- The Psychiatric Status Schedule (PSS) combines assessment of symptoms with assessment of social functioning (Spitzer *et al.*, 1970). It is also primarily a research instrument and is particularly useful in the assessment of less severely disabled people.
- Another type of assessment focuses on the nature and extent of particular impairments whose presence is suggested by psychiatric examination and which are thought to have implications for treatment and management. Negative symptoms of schizophrenia are an example; their differential diagnosis from depressive symptoms, side-effects of medication and features of behaviour thought to be associated with personality disorder or institutionalism can present problems.

The Scale for the Assessment of Negative Symptoms (SANS) was developed by Andreasen (1982) to overcome these diagnostic problems. It measures affective blunting or flattening, poverty of thought and speech, avolition, anhedonia and attentional difficulties. The ratings are based on direct observation and on reports from nurses and relatives as well as on self-reports.

- Rating scales which measure those impairments that have a direct, significant relationship with behaviour are particularly suited to practical rehabilitation assessments. Wing's Classification of Chronic Schizophrenia (1961) is a short scale that reliably rates the presence and degree of both positive and negative symptoms; it is easy to use and economical on time.

- The Manchester Scale (Krawiecka *et al.*, 1977), based on the Wing scale, has been widely used in the assessment of chronic symptoms; it also rates symptoms of depression and has the added advantage of rating drug side-effects if present. It is short, practical and easy to administer, and its sensitivity to change makes it valuable in assessing results of therapy and progress in rehabilitation over time.

(b) Assessment of physical disabilities

Physical ill-health and sensory impairments have far-reaching adverse effects on the mental state, social functioning and quality of life of people with psychiatric disability. Physical symptoms are sometimes disregarded, or they may receive insufficient attention, particularly in the case of community residents. In a large-scale community survey, Holmberg (1988) found that, in a population of 268 long-term outpatients, 65% had at least one physical health problem; significant conditions included hypertension, cardiovascular disease, respiratory and gastrointestinal disorders, diabetes, thyroid disorder, tardive dyskinesia and obesity. These conditions had a major negative impact on the respondents' quality of life and often interfered with rehabilitation efforts.

There are many factors that may contribute to the neglect of somatic disorders in this population. Some chronic, disabling physical illnesses develop slowly and may pass unnoticed; a proportion of people with psychiatric disability may not have sufficient knowledge or initiative to seek medical advice or may have difficulty in explaining their symptoms when they do; some believe that their complaints will either be thought by the doctor to be trivial or dismissed as part and parcel of their psychiatric disorder or evidence of drug side-effects. Rehabilitation professional staff need to be aware of these problems, to carry out preliminary physical assessments if appropriate and to facilitate suitable consultations. In carrying out assessments and reviews it is important to note the appearance of physical abnormalities and to follow up reports made by relatives, community nurses or workshop supervisors of observed physical difficulties such as breathlessness, poor eyesight, etc.

The side-effects of psychotropic drugs are worth special attention and appropriate checks should be routinely carried out. Apart from the regular laboratory tests when drugs such as lithium, anticonvulsants and some antipsychotic and antidepressant drugs are prescribed, evidence of extrapyramidal symptoms in those receiving antipsychotic medication should always be sought. The Abnormal Involuntary Movement Rating Scale (Guy, 1976) is often used in the assessment of symptoms of tardive dyskinesia (facial and oral movements, movements of neck, trunk, extremities and entire body); the presence and severity of these symptoms can be quickly rated but, because these symptoms tend to fluctuate, ratings should be made at regular intervals, preferably by the same observer.

(c) Assessment of social functioning

The assessment of the specifications of social functioning is central to every individual rehabilitation plan and it is the main basis for planning rehabilitation services. These assessments rely mainly on rating scales or schedules designed to measure social behaviour.

(d) Major reviews of social function assessment scales

In 1977, Hall published an analysis of five ward rating scales which were constructed to measure the social behaviour of long-stay hospital patients and which were in common use. He concluded that ratings should have a demonstrable association with reponse to treatment and that they should include the opinions of nurses and other carers and not just those of psychiatrists and psychologists, taking into account the effects of behaviour in the home and other community settings and not just in the hospital ward. He also reviewed 29 published ward rating scales (1980), according to five recommended criteria of acceptability that a potential user of any scale should apply.

1. The content of the scale has been selected on a rational basis.
2. The observation period on which ratings are based has been specified.
3. The scores are related to clearly defined norms.
4. The reliability of the scale has been assessed.
5. The validity of the scale has been assessed.

Descriptions of the rating setting, the rating procedure and the scale constructed should be given. Hall observed that most rating scales used in populations of long-term patients share similar practical characteristics, in that they require no equipment, scores are made directly from the response sheet, no special experience is required from the rater and, therefore, the choice of a particular scale tends to be based on balancing the value of the quantity and quality of information against the extra time and effort demanded from the rater and from the patient in making the assessments.

In practice, many rehabilitation services do not adhere to Hall's ideal; it is not uncommon, for example, for scales to be designed or modified, without applying strict criteria, to suit the purposes of day-to-day work in the light of clinical experience. Such initiatives, though unscientific, are understandable; it should be remembered that standard scales were often developed through trial and error.

Similar comments on the choice of scales were made by Weissman (1975), in a review of 15 scales designed to measure social adjustment, comprising the elements of social role performance, social supports, social attachments, social competence and social status.

In another review of 16 instruments considered to be suitable for measuring social functioning in rehabilitation, Wallace (1986) analysed each of the scales according to its content, format and psychometric characteristics, and discussed its advantages and disadvantages. He noted that the scales ranged from those that provide relatively global assessments of major life roles to those with more specific assessments of discrete behaviours, for example in the areas of personal hygiene and money management skills; this difference between the two types of assessment makes it difficult to integrate information across instruments and to compare the effectiveness of different rehabilitation procedures. Wallace also concluded that none of the reviewed instruments was wholly adequate for assessing functional living skills.

Since symptoms affect social functioning in varying degrees, the majority of scales used in rehabilitation practice tend to contain items which rate symptoms as well as items which rate social performance. Platt (1986), however, adopted the standpoint that there was a distinction between symptomatic behaviour, such as slowness or overactivity, and disturbance of social roles; it was his view that to evaluate the effectiveness of interventions, symptoms and social functioning behaviours should be independently rated. In this critical review, Platt examined the underlying concepts of seven social function scales; he classified them according to the norms that they used as yardsticks, as well as the dimensions of functioning that they measured, in assessing role performance. The content of social roles varies according to a variety of factors including age, sex, marital status, social class, race, etc; in addition, the norms used may be based on an ideal, a statistical average or the pre-illness behaviour of the individual. Platt concluded that the use of scales based on the concept of 'social performance', where behaviour is matched against cultural expectations of average functioning, is preferable to using 'social adjustment' scales, which tend to use ideal norms.

(e) Examples of rating scales

Wing's original work was the springboard for most social behaviour schedules in current use. His scale for measuring behaviour in chronic schizophrenia (1960) specifically assesses symptomatic behaviour; its two subscales measure deficits in behaviour, or social withdrawal (SW), and deviant or socially embarrassing behaviour (SEB). This scale is unsurpassed for its clarity, accuracy and ease of administration.

The **Nurses' Observation Scale for Inpatient Evaluation (NOSIE)** was developed by Honigfeld and Klett in 1965 and is still widely used. Although some of its items measure aspects of social performance – for example, personal neatness – most of the items rated reflected symptomatic behaviour in severely disabled patients.

The **Rehabilitation Evaluation of Hall and Baker – REHAB** (Baker and Hall, 1983) – was designed for the assessment of institutionalized patients. It measures difficult or embarrassing behaviour, as well as general social function behaviours. The scores are combined for five subscales (social activity, speech disturbance, speech skills, self-care skills and community skills) plus a total which includes a rating of overall functioning. It is simple to administer and is effective in measuring change when assessments are repeated. This instrument has been widely used to differentiate patients whose performance may enable them to live in community settings from those whose behaviour may prevent them from doing so, although doubts have been cast on the accuracy of these differentiations (Rowland, Perkins and Bennett, 1987; Conning and Brownlow, 1992). It is rather expensive to purchase.

The **Independent Living Skills Survey (ILSS)** designed by Wallace (1986) is a social adjustment questionnaire. Its 112 items cover the areas of eating, grooming, domestic activities, health care, money management, transportation, leisure activities and work; its two scales measure the frequency and the extent of problems over the range of behaviours. Its notable comprehensiveness is both an advantage and a disadvantage.

The **Morningside Rehabilitation Status Scale (MRSS)** was specifically designed for use in rehabilitation services (Affleck and McGuire, 1984). It is scored on four dimensions of dependence/independence, inactivity (occupation and leisure), social isolation/integration, and current symptoms and deviant behaviour; the scores are expressed as a profile of the dimensions, with a total score representing the overall level of functioning. It is easily administered by staff members who know the patient, and it requires no extensive training for its use. Apart from defining current levels of function and relating them to suitable, graded environmental settings, the scale is serviceable in measuring change following interventions. In practice, the measurements are likely to be more accurate in hospital populations than in community residents.

The **MRC Social Performance Schedule (SPS)** has been effectively used in research (Hurry and Sturt, 1981). It measures eight areas of social role performance (household management, employment, money management, child care, intimate relationships, social presentation of self and coping with emergencies). By defining performance in terms of the presence or absence of serious problems, the schedule avoids the use of ideal norms and it is particularly appropriate for the behaviour assessment of people with moderate psychiatric disability living in community settings.

A shorter **Social Behaviour Schedule (SBS)** was later developed (Wykes and Sturt, 1982) for the measurement of the range of behaviours found in social disablement, and it is especially suitable for surveying populations in hospital and community settings.

The **Social Functioning Scale (SFS)** is a new instrument designed by Birchwood *et al.* (1990) to assess social performance following family interventions. It is based on the WHO Disability Assessment Schedule (World Health Organisation, 1980); its ratings include scores for social engagement/withdrawal, interpersonal relationships, recreation, employment and independence. Its main interest lies in its intended application in the assessment of the efficacy of a specific intervention, but its ultimate value can only be determined after more extensive use.

The **Community Placement Questionnaire** has been specifically designed to aid planning for long-stay patients resident in hospitals scheduled for run-down or closure (Clifford *et al.*, 1991). In addition, this is a new instrument which needs to be tested over a period of time. It is aimed at assisting the planning of services rather than just looking at individuals.

The above examples illustrate some of the underlying concepts of the scales used in measuring social functioning, and some of the factors which might be considered when choosing scales for a particular purpose. The perfect instrument does not exist, and the choice of an assessment method will depend on the needs and orientation of the particular rehabilitation service and on the specific questions asked. Scales that rely more on observations than on self-reporting, that pay particular attention to performance rather than competence, or ability to perform a task, and about which psychometric data are available are to be preferred. An overriding consideration may well be the practicability and simplicity of application in day-to-day work.

3.2.2 ASSESSMENT OF RELATIONSHIPS

The growing literature on the powerful influence of family relationships and social networks in the course of rehabilitation has led to the development of a number of methods to evaluate their extent and quality, and to serve as a guide for interventions.

(a) Family assessment

Within a rehabilitation framework, family interventions have been shown to have positive effects on the disabled person and on the relatives; such interventions have to be based on the assessment of relevant family factors. In a review by Birley and Hudson (1982) these factors were summarized with reference to family influence on the person's mental state (the relationship between high expressed emotion (EE) levels and symptom relapse); family influence on the person's attitudes (aims, expectations and the sick role); the effect of family attitudes on the rehabilitation programme staff; and the effect of family influence on the person's financial rewards. Well-documented valid and reliable formal assessments are only available for the measurement of EE (Brown and Rutter, 1966) and even in its shortened form this method is time-consuming and requires fairly intensive training. The assessment of these factors, therefore tends to rely mostly on informal observation.

From another perspective, schedules used to measure family burden, both objective and subjective, can give an indication of the level of disability of the disabled member and may point to specific areas where family support is needed.

(b) Other social networks

Studies carried out in hospitals have revealed the existence of various relationship patterns among long-stay patients (Harries, Frois and Healey, 1984) and a more recent observational study led to the development of the Social Network Schedule (SNS) by Dunn *et al.* (1990), which categorizes the types of behaviour in relation to social contacts (see also section 5.3). About one third of the study population were 'asocial', with a low quality and quantity of contacts; this group was severely disabled. These findings have implications for service organization and planning: the process of hospital closure often involves the selective discharge of the more socially able, leaving behind the least able and 'asocial', who may be further disadvantaged and even less likely to form viable social networks when eventually discharged from hospital. This may be mitigated by planning and creating additional social support, for example through day care, for those who are unable to develop social networks by themselves.

3.2.3 ASSESSING THE QUALITY OF LIFE

The classical three-hospital study by Wing and Brown (1970) has shown that a rich, stimulating environment has significantly positive effects on negative impairments of schizophrenia, while high levels of emotional stimulation in some families have been shown to have a direct relationship with positive symptom relapse and depression (Vaughan and Leff, 1976). One aspect of the recognition of the importance of the environment has been a growing interest in quality of life studies. Malm, May and Dencker (1981) have suggested that the assessment of quality of life comprises a subjective judgement of the environment and objectively measured environmental conditions; it is therefore a simultaneous evaluation of satisfaction and of living conditions. Such assessments usually consist of checklists, with indicators of the quality of medical care, human relationships, material conditions, communication and transport services, open and sheltered employment, safety, knowledge and inner minor experiences.

Lehman, Ward and Linn (1982), whose work has been influential in this field, attempted to dissect eight areas of quality of life: living situation, family relationships, social relationships, work, leisure activities, finance, safety and health. There are difficult methodological issues in such assessments. The 'objective' aspects are based on norms and baselines which must vary according to cultural expectations, prior experiences and individual perceptions – in short, they have the same pitfalls as most social adjustment measures; the 'subjective' aspects, as in consumer surveys, have the drawback of being inevitably coloured and highly influenced by the current mental state.

Another important aspect was highlighted by Thapa and Rowland (1989) in a study aimed at the specific perspectives of long-term care in which they developed an instrument to assess the quality of life as part of the rehabilitation programme. A comparison between staff and patient perceptions of the quality of life across several domains disclosed significant differences in several areas, including leisure, law, and safety and health. The implications are that staff should be cautious in drawing conclusions about factors that may improve the quality of life. However, such checklists are useful in focusing attention on the environment and they can yield useful common-sense information.

3.2.4 WORK ASSESSMENT

The main objective of rehabilitation work assessment is to enable decisions to be made on future work placements; it therefore encompasses the measurement of physical and psychological limitations, aptitudes and interests, as well as the potential for education and training (Roberts, 1970). It takes into account the type of work involved and the environmental factors of work settings.

(a) Past performance

The first element which work assessments address is past performance; it is vital to have accurate information on educational attainments and previous employment records. These historical facts are highly relevant to work rehabilitation outcome; people with an early onset of illness and long periods of hospitalization may find extreme difficulty in settling into a regular work routine since they never acquire a 'work personality'. Those who were unemployed for more than two years prior to hospital admission, and those with a poor record of past occupational stability, also have a less favourable outlook when employment is considered (Watts and Bennett, 1977). These factors may therefore affect the type and duration of work rehabilitation interventions.

(b) Mental state and symptoms

Although the individual's mental state is an important element of the work assessment, symptomatic behaviour, rather than symptoms *per se*, is more relevant; a person who retains an elaborate, but encapsulated, delusional system can function satisfactorily at work, while the performance of another who has no detectable florid symptoms can be consistently poor because of slowness or lowered drive.

(c) Social circumstances

Social circumstances such as the type of living accommodation, financial state and social supports outside work can have significant effects on work performance. The assessment of these aspects, therefore, is pertinent.

(d) Work rating scales

Van Allen and Loeber (1972) critically reviewed a number of published work rating scales designed for hospital populations. The catalogue of deficiencies which they found in many included inadequate description of the nature of the work setting and types of patient population, as well as a dearth of normative data. They classified the items commonly found in the scales under five main headings: 'work personality', work competence, social competence, psychiatric symptoms and more general factors; the majority of the scales emphasized the importance of work competence over social competence and 'work personality'; psychiatric symptomatology was considered to be less important than other factors as an indicator of work performance. One of the perennial difficulties in work assessment is rater bias; some assessors are more lenient than others in rating work performance, and this is usually more apparent when the rated items are related to pay. Remuneration, in real life, is not a good indicator of performance although, theoretically, it should be.

Work rating scales have many features in common; their main items tend to emphasize both instrumental performance, or competence, and social behaviour. A good example is the St Wulstan Scale (Cheadle *et al.*, 1967), which was based on the assessment forms used in the Industrial Rehabilitation Units (IRUs) of the British Ministry of Labour and on an unpublished Netherne Hospital scale. It was simple to use in a variety of work situations and easy to administer by members of various professional disciplines; seven of its 15 items rated instrumental performance such as speed, persistence and manual skills and eight rated attitudes and social behaviour, including eagerness to work, positive attitude to supervision and relationships. Similarly, the Griffiths Scale (Griffiths, 1973) rated both task competence and social behaviour and attitudes.

In their guidelines for current users of work assessments and for future construction of scales, Van Allen and Loeber suggested that the scales should include:

1. descriptions of the populations for which the scales are to be used, their demographic characteristics and their previous work histories;
2. defined 'norms' for rating;
3. descriptions of the work setting, working hours and pay rates;
4. a system of feedback of the results to the worker and to staff members concerned with aspects of his or her case.

(e) Psychometric tests

Intelligence is not a predictor of either work performance or future employability, but it can predict the choice of the level of job.

Assessment of personality characteristics, on the whole, is also a poor predictor of future work performance. Tests of vocational aptitudes, for example, the General Aptitude Test Battery (United States Department of Labor, 1965) do not predict employability; they are of value, however, in exploring skills and training potential and providing a focus of vocational counselling. Interest inventories, such as the Weingarten Picture Interest Inventory (Weingarten, 1958), are useful in exploring an individual's interests and for comparability with skills.

(f) Work sampling

Work abilities may be assessed on real or simulated samples of actual jobs, using the same materials, tools and equipment that the jobs normally require. The assessment entails specific ratings for dexterity, productivity and time limits. For work sampling to be of real value, factors such as relationships with workmates and supervisors, punctuality, appropriate dress and general presentation of the self, behaviour related to lunch and tea breaks, etc. have to be taken into consideration.

(g) Work experience

The results of assessments carried out in hospitals or community workshops, however realistically the work and the environment may be structured, cannot confidently be extrapolated to open employment; generalization of behaviour is notoriously difficult, so that the transfer of learned work skills from a sheltered, therapeutic situation to a job may be a veritable quantum leap. Work experience is a try-out in a real work situation with real work; the worker is placed, for example, within an industrial firm where he or she is expected to work like everyone else, subject to the same employment discipline, while still in receipt of state benefit for a limited period of acclimatization and assessment. This has the added advantage of involving the employer in the assessment without extra cost and of giving the worker additional insight into his or her abilities and limitations.

3.2.5 ASSESSMENT OF SERVICES

A fundamental aspect of the evaluation or assessment of rehabilitation services is the measurement of their adequacy to achieve their objectives. Evaluation is not only concerned with outcome (Chapter 8) but also with the processes involved in meeting the objectives. Holland (1983), for example, stated that evaluation determines the effectiveness, efficiency and acceptability of planned interventions in achieving stated objectives. The information provided from evaluation will guide the service's future policy and practice. An evaluation contains seeds of change; the service has to respond to changes in its population, but it has to continue serving its specific client group. There is a common tendency to drift towards serving the more able, 'rewarding' clients; hostels developed for people with severe disabilities, for example, may start rejecting residents who are not sociable and community teams may begin to take on 'acute patients' in order to 'keep up interest'.

(a) Process of evaluation

There are three stages in the process of evaluation.

Deciding what to evaluate. The first step is to determine the objectives and the philosophy of the service. A service whose aims lack clarity is difficult to evaluate and its delivery of care is likely to be unsatisfactory. The philosophy has to be translated into concrete, measurable terms. Evaluation has to be comprehensive at three levels: that of the individuals and their problems, that of the most effective treatments and that of the service delivery (Wing, 1972, 1987).

Carrying out the evaluation. The methodology chosen for evaluation must be appropriate so that it answers the questions posed. If the purpose is to influence policy in the immediate future, for example, it is inappropriate to employ research designs which would take a long time to set up and carry out. It is essential to be mindful of the time and resources available, as well as of the cost. Evaluations must not impede staff from carrying out their duties nor patients from receiving the care to which they are entitled.

Using the information. Although satisfying curiosity and academic interest is important (Wing, 1987), evaluation should ultimately influence practice and generate further evaluation. Since its results could influence the shape of the service, the information gained should be clearly documented and fed back to managers and planners.

Quantity of service. A rehabilitation service comprises a dedicated team of staff and chains of residential, day and other community services. Methods of evaluating quantity of service rely on descriptive statistics – for example the number of beds in use per 100 000 of the population, the ratio of day places to beds and the number of hostel places – and on case registers (Wing, 1972). Descriptive statistics are often related to norms or to minimum standards, bearing in mind that these are not absolute and that they are determined also by local conditions and population characteristics; Hirsch (1988), for instance, showed that there is a significant association between social deprivation and psychiatric morbidity, which has major implications for planning levels of provision (Chapter 7).

Quality of service.   This is much more difficult to measure; apart from the physical conditions of the provisions, staffing levels and staff attitudes, the prevailing atmosphere of the various settings, the relationships within the service and between the service and other organizations are all decisive determinants of quality. Wing and Freudenberg (1961), for example, showed that the quality of supervision in a hospital workshop had significant effects on the behaviour of severely disabled patients. Similarly, the incidence and severity of symptomatic behaviour of such patients were correlated with the prevalent social environment of the hospital (Wing and Brown, 1970). The course and outcome of work rehabilitation may also be influenced by other environmental factors; in an industrial rehabilitation unit, the enthusiastic and confidence-building attitudes of the reference group positively contributed to the rehabilitation outcome of people with moderate disability (Wing, 1966). In another study, Floyd (1984) demonstrated that people disabled by schizophrenia were more likely to maintain employment where the work environment had a high degree of objective quality, including the provision of clear feedback on performance.

(b) Assessment methods

The way services have been evaluated has been influenced by the prevailing social climate. In the 1960s and 1970s, evaluation tended to target aspects of institutional care which had come under criticism (Moos, 1969; King, Raynes and Tizard, 1971). Since the early 1980s there has been a shift, potentiated by health service managers, towards assessing the totality of services and their performance.

Assessments which have been developed to evaluate health services are based on measuring three important variables:

- identification of specific problems which cause social disablement;
- identification of methods likely to solve or ameliorate these problems;
- application of appropriate interventions, by appropriate agents, in service settings and measuring the outcome in terms of success in solving the problems (Wing, 1990).

This approach, therefore, diagnoses the disabilities, specifies forms of help such as training, medication and support, and also highlights elements of service which are needed. An estimate can then be made of the service's provisions and gaps, which will assist future planning. This exciting development in service evaluation is still comparatively new and, although it is a research method, its wider application may prove to be valuable in service work.

REFERENCES

Affleck, J.W. and McGuire, R.J. (1984) The measurement of psychiatric rehabilitation status: a review of the needs and a new scale. *British Journal of Psychiatry*, **145**, 517–525.

Andreasen, N. (1982) Negative symptoms in schizophrenia: definition and reliability. *Archives of General Psychiatry*, **39**, 784–788.

Baker, R. and Hall, N.J. (1983) *Rehabilitation Evaluation of Hall and Baker (REHAB)*, Vine Publishing, Aberdeen.

Birchwood, M., Smith, J., Cochrane, R. *et al.* (1990) The Social Functioning Scale: the development and validation of a new scale of social adjustment for use in family intervention programmes with schizophrenia patients. *British Journal of Psychiatry*, **157**, 853–859.

Birley, J. and Hudson, B. (1983) The family, the social network and rehabilitation, in *Theory and Practice of Psychiatric Rehabilitation*, (eds F.N. Watts and D.H. Bennett), John Wiley & Sons, Chichester.

Bradshaw, J. (1972) The concept of social need. *New Society*, **30**, 640–643.

Brewin, C.R., Wing, J.K. Mangen, S.P. *et al.* (1987) Principles and practice of measuring needs in the long term mentally ill: the MRC Needs for Care Assessment. *Psychological Medicine*, **17**, 971–981.

Brown, G.W. and Rutter, M. (1966) The measurement of family activities and relationships: a methodological study. *Human Relation*, **19**, 241–263.

Cheadle, A.J., Cushing, D., Drew, C.D.A. and Morgan, R. (1967) The measurement of the work performance of psychiatric patients. *British Journal of Psychiatry*, **113**, 841–846.

Clifford, P., Charman, A., Webb, Y. *et al.* (1991) Planning for community care: the Community Placement Questionnaire. *British Journal of Clinical Psychology*, **30**, 193–211.

Conning, A.M. and Brownlow, J. (1992) Determining suitability of placement for long-stay psychiatric inpatients. *Hospital and Community Psychiatry*, **43**(7), 709–712.

Dunn, M., O'Driscoll, C., Dayson, D. *et al.* (1990) The TAPS Project: 4. An observational study of the social life of long-stay patients. *British Journal of Psychiatry*, **57**, 842–848.

Ekdawi, M.Y. (1990) The components of psychiatric rehabilitation services, in *International Perspectives in Schizophrenia*, (ed. M Weller), John Libby, London.

Falloon, I.R.H. (1990) Family management of schizophrenia, in *International Perspectives in Schizophrenia*, (ed. M. Weller), John Libby, London.

Floyd, M. (1984) The employment problems of people disabled by schizophrenia. *Journal of Social and Occupational Medicine*, **34**, 93–95.

Griffiths, R.D.P. (1973) A standardised assessment of the work behaviour of psychiatric patients. *British Journal of Psychiatry*, **123**, 403–408.

Guy, W. (1976) *ECDEU Manual for Psychopharmacology*, DHEW, Washington, DC.

Hall, N.J. (1976) Assessment procedures used in studies on long-stay patients: a survey of papers published in the British Journal of Psychiatry. *British Journal of Psychiatry*, **135**, 330–335.

Hall, N.J. (1977) The content of ward rating scales for long-stay patients. *British Journal of Psychiatry*, **130**, 287–293.

Hall, N,.J. (1980) Ward rating scales for long-stay patients: a review. *Psychological Medicine*, **10**, 277–288.

Hall, N.J. (1981) Psychological assessment, in *Handbook of Psychiatric Rehabilitation Practice*, (eds J.K. Wing and B. Morris), Oxford University Press, Oxford.

Harries, C., Frois, M. and Healey, J. (1984) 'The hidden society': the practical use of multi-dimensional scaling to illuminate the pattern of relationships between long-stay psychiatric residents. *Journal of Advanced Nursing*, **9**, 619–625.

Hirsch, S. (1988) *Psychiatric Beds and Resources: Factors in Financing Bed Use and Service Planning*, Gaskell (Royal College of Psychiatrists), London.

Holland, W.W. (1983) *Evaluation of Health Care*, Oxford Medical Publications, Oxford.

Holmberg, S. (1988) *The Status of Physical Health in the Long-term Mentally Ill: Psychiatric Record Review of 268 Patients*. Abstracts of the IV International Congress on Rehabilitation Psychiatry, Orebro, Sweden.

Honigfeld, G. and Klett, C.J. (1965) The nurses' observation scale for in-patient evaluation. *Journal of Clinical Psychology*, **21**, 65–71.

Hurry, J. and Sturt, E. (1981) Social performance in a population sample: relation to psychiatric symptoms, in *What is a Case?*, (eds J.K. Wing, P. Bebbington and L.N. Robbins) Grant McIntyre, London.

Kendell, R.E., Everitt, B., Cooper, J.E. *et al.* (1968) The reliability of 'Present State Examination'. *Social Psychiatry*, **3**, 123–129.

King, R.D., Raynes, N.V. and Tizard, J. (1971) *Patterns of Residential Care*, Routledge and Kegan Paul, London.

Krawiecka, M., Goldberg, D. and Vaughan, M. (1977) A standardised assessment scale for rating chronic psychiatric patients. *Acta Psychiatrica Scandinavica*, **55**, 299–308.

Lehman, A.F., Ward, N.C. and Linn, L.S. (1982) Chronic mental patients: the quality of life issue. *American Journal of Psychiatry*, **139**, 1271–1276.

Malm, U., May, P.R.A. and Dencker, S.J. (1981) Evaluation of the quality of life of schizophrenic outpatients: a checklist. *Schizophrenia Bulletin*, **7**, 477–485.

Moos, R. (1969) *Ward Atmosphere Scale Preliminary Manual*, Social Ecology Laboratory, Stanford University, California.

Platt, S. (1986) Evaluating social functioning. A critical review of scales and underlying concepts, in *The Psychopharmacology and Treatment of Schizophrenia*, (eds P.B. Bradley and S. Hirsch), Oxford University Press, Oxford.

Roberts, C.L. (1970) Definitions, objectives and goals in work evaluation. *Journal of Rehabilitation*, **36**, 12–15.

Rowland, L., Perkins, R. and Bennett, D. (1987) Planning community services for the long-term disabled: the Maudsley experience. Unpublished manuscript.

Spitzer, R.L., Endicott, J., Fleiss, J.L. and Cohen, J. (1970) The Psychiatric Status Schedule: a technique for evaluating psychopathology and impairment of role functioning. *Archives of General Psychiatry*, **23**, 41–55.

Thapa, K. and Rowland, L.A. (1989) Quality of life perspectives in long-term care: staff and patient perceptions. *Acta Psychiatrica Scandinavica*, **80**, 267–271.

United States Department of Labor (1965) *General Aptitude Test Battery*, United States Department of Labor, Manpower Administration, Bureau of Employment Security, Washington, DC.

Van Allen, R. and Loeber, R. (1972) Work assessment of psychiatric patients: a critical review of published scales. *Canadian Journal of Behavioural Science*, **4**, 101–117.

Vaughan, C.E. and Leff, J.P. (1976) The influence of family and social factors on the course of psychiatric symptoms: a comparison of schizophrenic and depressed neurotic patients. *British Journal of Psychiatry*, **129**, 125–137.

Wallace, C.J. (1986) Functional assessment in rehabilitation. *Schizophrenia Bulletin*, **4**, 604–630.

Watts, F.N. and Bennett, D.H. (1977) Previous occupational stability as a predictor of employment after psychiatric rehabilitation. *Psychological Medicine*, **7**, 763–767.

Weingarten, K.P. (1958) *Weingarten Picture Interest Inventory*, McGraw-Hill, California.

Weissman, M.M. (1975) The assessment of social adjustment. *Archives of General Psychiatry*, **32**, 358–365.

Wing, J.K. (1960) The measurement of behaviour in chronic schizophrenia. *Acta Psychiatrica Scandinavica*, **35**, 245–254.

Wing, J.K. (1961) A simple and reliable classification of chronic schizophrenia. *Journal of Mental Science*, **107**, 862–875.

Wing, J.K. (1966) Social and psychological changes in a rehabilitation unit. *Social Psychiatry*, **1**, 21–28.

Wing, J.K. (1972) Principles of evaluation, in *Evaluating a Community Psychiatric Service* (eds J.K. Wing and A.M. Hailey) Oxford University Press, Oxford.

Wing, J. (1987) Evaluative research: an underpopulated science, in *New Directions in Mental Health Evaluation*, (eds I. Marks, J. Connolly and M. Muikin), Institute of Psychiatry, London.

Wing, J.K. (1990) Planning and evaluating health and social services for people with a long-term psychiatric disorder, in *The Public Health Impact of Mental Disorder*, (eds D. Goldberg and D. Tantum), Hogrefe & Huber, Toronto.

Wing, J.K. and Brown, G.W. (1970) Institutionalism and Schizophrenia, Cambridge University Press, Cambridge.

Wing, J.K. and Freudenberg, R.K. (1961) The response of severely ill chronic schizophrenic patients to social stimulation. *American Journal of Psychiatry*, **118**, 311–322.

World Health Organisation (1980) *International Classification of Impairments, Disabilities and Handicaps*, World Health Organisation, Geneva.

Wykes, T. and Sturt, E. (1982) A hostel ward for 'new' long-stay patients: an evaluative study of a 'ward-in-a-house', in *Long Term Community Care: Experience in a London Borough*, (ed. J.K. Wing), Psychological Medicine Monograph Supplement 2, Cambridge University Press, Cambridge.

Rehabilitation
interventions

4

4.1 MEDICATION

The aims of prescribed drugs in rehabilitation are to relieve and
control symptoms and to prevent relapse. The heterogeneity of
presentation, course of long-term illness and diversity of individual
responses to medication demand careful and often time-consuming
assessments and monitoring. It is accepted that medication primarily
targeted at symptoms, rather than at diagnostic categories, is the most
profitable prescribing approach (Johnstone, Crow and Firth, 1988) and
that a single pharmacological agent cannot be expected to treat all the
manifestations of a psychosis (Donaldson, Gelenberg and Baldessarini,
1983). In the long term, the effort to prevent relapse of acute symptoms
once they are controlled justifies months of considered trial of drugs
(Crammer and Heine, 1991) since the consequences of relapse are
disastrous.

While it is preferable to avoid polypharmacy (the prescription of
several drugs together) as much as possible (Holloway, 1988), many
patients need to have combined medication at times. Thus, a patient
with a diagnosis of schizophrenia may be prescribed antidepressants
in addition to maintenance antipsychotic drugs. Regimens which
rigidly 'rationalize' polypharmacy at all costs, for example by changing
over from combinations of oral and injectable depot medication to
equivalent doses of depot alone, may result in increased relapse rates
(Soni et al., 1992).

4.1.1 MAINTENANCE MEDICATION

The value of maintenance medication in limiting the incidence of
symptom exacerbation and recurrence in schizophrenia and severe
affective disorders has been established and well documented (Leff

and Wing, 1971, Quitkin *et al.*, 1981, Coppen and Abou-Saleh, 1988, Johnson *et al.*, 1983). It is also generally held that social and psychological factors, such as some life events and high levels of expressed emotion, are likely to precipitate relapse (Birley and Brown, 1970, Leff and Vaughan, 1980) and that the risk of relapse is magnified in the absence of the protective effects of maintenance medication. Therefore, a combination of psychosocial approaches and medication achieves the best rehabilitation results (Hogarty, 1984); both types of intervention should be viewed as having supplementary and not competing roles (May, 1976).

The use of drugs in long-term management is not to be lightly undertaken; their actions, limitations and side-effects should be thoroughly familiar to the prescriber, and careful evaluation of the risk–benefit ratio in each case is essential (Johnson, 1990). This is particularly pertinent when disabling and distressing symptoms persist despite an appropriate type and dosage of medication. It has been estimated that about 25% of people with schizophrenia are treatment-resistant in terms of their poor response to conventional antipsychotic drugs; in such cases, it is important to resist the temptation to resort to 'alternative therapies' of no proven value (Christison, Darrell and Wyatt, 1991) that may cause additional disability.

Apart from the type of maintenance medication and its dose, the route of administration can be crucial. Oral medication has the advantage of being more acceptable to many patients than injections; however, it carries the risks of inconsistency and overdose. The commonly held belief that oral medication is short-acting, allowing flexibility in varying the dosage, is incorrect; active metabolites of orally administered antipsychotic drugs tend to remain in the body for weeks or months after they are discontinued (Johnson, 1990). Depot medication ensures more constant drug blood levels at lower doses and it also gives a more accurate picture of the response to the drug. In addition, there is evidence that patients receiving it are less likely to relapse.

Clinical experience has shown that some patients whose symptoms are successfully controlled for many years relapse when maintenance medication is discontinued. In an excellent review based on long-term studies, Johnson (1990) concluded that the duration of long-term medication remains uncertain; however, even after 5 years from the last episode of illness, 80% of patients with a diagnosis of schizophrenia relapse when medication is discontinued. There are no known criteria which determine the 20% who can safely stop the medication.

In prescribing maintenance medication, three principles should be borne in mind.

- Regular assessments of the mental state should be carried out, even when it has remained stable for a long time; detection and treatment of early signs of psychotic relapse carry a better prognosis. There are also high morbidity rates in long-term illness due to depression; care must always be taken during the assessments not to miss depressive symptoms, however low-key their presentation.
- The clinician must always be vigilant in considering the prevailing psychosocial factors, as well as the current symptoms; they are often interlinked.
- Prompt diagnosis of side-effects is essential, although some may be difficult to treat and a balance has sometimes to be struck between the benefits of a drug and its unwanted effects. Various strategies have been proposed to minimize the long-term side-effects of antipsychotic drugs. Intermittent medication and 'drug holidays' have not been shown to reduce their incidence; very low dose medication, on balance, probably increases the risk of relapse; the advantages of individualized, flexible low dosage are debatable. The clinician may opt for prescribing one of the 'new generation' antipsychotic drugs in some instances. In deciding on an optimal medication, in all cases, there is no substitute for making individually based judgements.

4.1.2 NON-COMPLIANCE

Whenever a drug fails to achieve the desired therapeutic effect, one of the questions to be asked is whether it had been taken as prescribed. The term 'compliance' has unfortunate connotations of passive obedience; adherence to an agreed drug regime largely depends on the **involvement** of the patient – it is an area where patient empowerment is both important and rewarding. The extent of non-compliance is difficult to measure; it has been widely reported in many medical conditions, in inpatients as well as outpatients and during both short-term and long-term courses of medication. It has been estimated that up to 60% of people with a diagnosis of schizophrenia who live in the community are, at least episodically, non-compliant (Van Putten, 1974). Given the prophylactic significance of maintenance medication, it is vital to enlist the patient's cooperation; therefore, it is important to be aware of the issues which have a bearing on the acceptance of and adherence to prescribed drugs.

- There is a natural expectation that medication will relieve symptoms; once relief is experienced, there is a tendency to stop taking it or to forget. Although forgetting may be due to 'unintentional' risk-taking, it is often genuine, particularly when regimes are complicated and when they do not easily fit in with the patient's daily routine.

When a person feels well, it is difficult to continue with prophylactic medication especially when symptoms do not recur for long periods of time. It is even more difficult if symptoms re-emerge in spite of compliance; Waters and Northover (1965) showed that, in some instances, non-compliance follows rather than precedes recurrence.

- Psychotropic medication, in particular, is often perceived as stigmatizing and as a reminder of past illness. The individual taking it may feel diminished as a person, lacking in self-control; moral and religious scruples may also be involved. These factors were well illustrated in Perceval's nineteenth-century account (Bateson, 1961). During his psychotic illness, Perceval found it difficult to reconcile taking the healer's medicine with his wish to rely on God and on his own will-power; he eventually compromised by taking half the prescribed dose. It should also be remembered that many people find it disagreeable, in the case of maintenance depot medication, to be repeatedly injected.
- In addition to the unpleasant side-effects caused by some drugs, fears surrounding long-term harm and of addiction, which are sometimes aroused by media publicity, frequently deter adherence to medication.
- Poor fluctuating insight, which commonly occurs in psychotic states, is a major contributory factor to non-compliance.
- For those who are not exempt from prescription charges under welfare benefits rules, the expenditure on drugs can be an enormous budgetary item which they can ill-afford.

4.1.3 IMPROVING COMPLIANCE

Labelled drug packaging, the so-called compliance aids, are of limited value, particularly for people with cognitive impairments. There are two main rehabilitation approaches to improve adherence to medication, and both are often concurrently used.

Behavioural training in medication management relies on education in the effects and side-effects of drugs; the 'insurance policy' rationale for maintenance medication is repeatedly explained to the patient and to the relatives who, at the same time, are encouraged to voice their anxieties and to negotiate appropriate changes with the prescribing clinician (Liberman and Evans, 1985). The patient takes charge of the medication, so that monitored self-medication progresses, for example, from daily to weekly or monthly prescriptions. Feedback and positive reinforcement are essential in maintaining this learning process.

Counselling   aims at fairly fundamental changes in negative attitudes to medication through exploring and understanding the patient's feelings, beliefs and views. Since 'knowledge is a prerequisite of behaviour change' (Miller, Donegan and Curran, 1990), adequate and unambiguous information about medication is the essential first step. The assistance of the pharmacist in conveying such information is invaluable, and so is concise written material and information packs. Work in other specialized fields, such as AIDS counselling, has also shown that the ability to receive, retain and profit from information, so that risk behaviours are minimized, must go hand in hand with training in social skills (Higgins *et al.*, 1988); to be effective, therefore, information has to be given within the context of a comprehensive rehabilitation package. Apart from individual counselling, group counselling, which promotes the peer group's values and expectations and where the individual has the chance of benefiting from others' experiences, can be effective (Kelly and St Lawrence, 1990). During counselling sessions, it is best to avoid excessive 'fear messages'; the relationship between fear of illness and cigarette smoking, for example, is highly complex and inordinate fear may induce a sense of despair which, in turn, perpetuates risk behaviour.

There are important factors which improve the acceptability of maintenance medication. Continuity of care, which involves good relationships and facilitates easy communications between patient and prescriber, augments the chances of acceptance (Davis and Fallowfield, 1991). The organization of follow-up outpatient clinics is highly relevant. In an interesting study where levels of compliance were compared in five clinics, it was clearly shown that they correlated strongly with organizational differences; the most successful clinic retained three times as many people in treatment as the least successful. Significant factors for success included a team approach, with easy access to the team members, as well as frequent medication counselling (Attwood and Beck, 1985). Clinics which specialize in long-term care have greater compliance success than general psychiatry clinics and general practice surgeries (Coppen and Abou-Saleh, 1988). Regular attendance for treatment is more prevalent in clinics whose atmosphere is informal and welcoming and where waiting time is minimal. The time and venue of appointments should not inconvenience the patient (Liberman and Evans, 1985). Non-attendance should be quickly investigated, and assertive outreach and home visits may then prove to be necessary. As a rule, a patient who identifies with the clinic's client group, who enjoys the social aspects of the visit to the clinic and whose attendance is positively reinforced, is less likely to drop out.

In summary, long-term maintenance medication is one of the most important interventions within a rehabilitation package. It poses many challenges for the clinicians, the patients and the organization. An understanding of its benefits and its limitations, as well as of the factors which influence adherence to the treatment plan, has to be a joint, collaborative effort aimed at maintaining good health.

4.2 BEHAVIOURAL APPROACHES

One of the most valuable combinations which a clinical psychologist can make to a rehabilitation service is to bring a way of thinking based on theories of learning. Behavioural approaches have had a part to play in patient care throughout the history of rehabilitation, despite behaviourism's traditional focus on anxiety-based disorders such as phobias. Over the years, the application of behavioural techniques within long-term care has expanded and has been enhanced by the influence of cognitive approaches. Some of these applications will be examined below.

4.2.1 TOKEN ECONOMY PROGRAMMES

Token economy programmes (TEPs) were introduced in the 1960s and 1970s for the treatment of people with chronic schizophrenia living on the back wards of psychiatric asylums (Gripp and Magaro, 1974; Kazkin, 1978). In the decade prior to this, Goffman (1961) and Barton (1959) had criticized the regimes of the asylums and pointed out that many of the patients' symptoms were caused by what went on within the asylums, rather than by the mental illnesses themselves. This having been pointed out, there were two possible responses: close the asylums or improve what was taking place within them. As the asylums were not going to shut overnight, it was necessary to find ways of improving life for the residents, both by improving the social environment which indirectly increased patients' levels of functioning (Wing and Brown, 1970), and by carrying out interventions which were aimed directly at changing the patients' behaviour. It was here that token economy programmes played their part (Allyon and Azrin, 1968).

For each patient taking part in a TEP, clearly identifiable behavioural goals were set, such as getting out of bed in the morning before a specified time. The achievement of each goal was rewarded with a token, which was given immediately. These tokens could be exchanged at a later point in time, and at an agreed exchange rate, for other rewards such as sweets or cigarettes. It was common for a whole ward to be operating in this fashion, although the targeted behaviours were usually chosen individually for each patient. Although TEPs were very popular in the 1970s, this popularity has now declined, but it is not uncommon for individual patients to have behaviour management programmes (section 4.2.2).

The development of TEPs, and the research which they generated, helped to emphasize the importance of the social environment for patients. For example, Hall, Baker and Hutchinson (1977) demonstrated that the improvements in patients' functioning brought about by TEPs were the result not of the programmed rewards themselves but of the social reward which came with them, in the form of praise from, and pleasant interaction with, the staff. In a much larger study, Paul and Lentz (1977) showed that a social learning environment based around TEPs was superior to traditional hospital environments and social milieu environments, in terms both of increasing patients' adaptive functioning and decreasing unusual behaviours. The benefits derived not just from the TEPs themselves, but from the enhanced interpersonal communication and increased shared activities which went with them. It was the non-specific factors about TEPs which worked, rather than the programme rewards themselves (Tantum, 1992).

4.2.2 MANAGING DIFFICULT BEHAVIOUR

Sometimes patients in rehabilitation services present staff with the problem of managing their difficult behaviour. Examples might be: unacceptable and antisocial behaviour, such as making unwanted sexual advances; abusive or aggressive behaviour, such as verbal outbursts or threatening behaviour; or pestering people for money, cigarettes and so on. Difficult behaviours such as these pose particular problems in a rehabilitation setting for several reasons.

Firstly, because the care of such patients is long-term, staff can feel so worn down and irritated by having to cope with a difficult customer day after day that they begin to dislike or fear the patient, making any form of appropriate intervention difficult or unlikely. Secondly, if one of the aims for the patient is that he or she should be maintained without an inpatient admission to hospital, for as long as possible, such antisocial behaviour is a far greater barrier to successful placement than his or her ability to carry out daily living skills (Hill, 1988; Waismann, 1988; Conning and Brownlow, 1992). Thirdly, the trend for dispersing and fragmenting rehabilitation services means that staff often find themselves working alone or in small groups, such as one 'housekeeper' looking afer eight residents in a hostel. In such a situation, if the member of staff feels frightened by, or unable to cope with, someone's difficult behaviour, then it is the patient who will suffer, by having to leave.

Behavioural techniques can play an invaluable part in managing difficult behaviour. Where a person cannot internally generate and maintain appropriate limits on his or her behaviour because of cognitive or emotional disabilities, then it is important that they are provided for in the outside world (Perkins and Dilks, 1992). A behaviour management programme can be an appropriate way of providing such limits. Some of the principles, and possible hurdles, involved will be illustrated by a case study.

Case study: Fred

Fred was a man in his late fifties who lived on his own in a small and barely furnished local authority flat. He attended the local rehabilitation day unit on a daily basis, including weekends, and was one of the first to arrive and the last to leave. Over several months, Fred's behaviour in the day unit had become more and more irritating and was complained about by staff and residents alike. The nursing staff asked for help from the psychologist in managing his behaviour.

The first task was to define the behaviour which other people found unacceptable. This was important so that Fred would know what it was he was doing which upset other people and so that staff could be clear about the behaviour that they were trying to change. Fred's unacceptable behaviours were defined as follows:

- taking other people's food in the canteen;
- demanding meals to which he was not entitled;
- touching people in an inappropriate, but non-sexual way;
- using threatening behaviour, e.g. shouting and demanding things;
- using violence;
- being sexually disinhibited, e.g. by exposing himself;
- making indecent assaults, e.g. touching someone else sexually when it was not wanted;
- making unwanted sexual propositions.

Definitions of the unacceptable behaviours were obtained by talking to members of staff and by observing Fred's behaviour and the reactions of others to it. These observations also showed that staff and patients rarely spoke to Fred other than when they were shouting at him in response to his behaviour. In behavioural terms, Fred was rewarded for his unacceptable behaviour by being noticed by other people, while he was largely ignored the rest of the time. Although 'being noticed' usually meant being shouted at, Fred had such an engaging smile and infectious laugh that it was difficult not to be drawn in to his laughter.

The next step was to find a suitable reward for Fred when he behaved in an acceptable manner. He was already provided with an evening meal by the day unit, but staff who knew him well were in agreement that a midday meal would be an appropriate reward for him. Fred rarely cooked for himself at home, had refused to be trained in cooking skills at the unit on many occasions and frequently tried to sneak in for a lunch to which he was not entitled. However, as Fred's behaviour appeared to be aimed at getting people to take notice of him, it was important to build in some other rewards for appropriate behaviour. The following actions were agreed on.

- The charge nurse would go with Fred to his flat once a fortnight to help him clean up. Keeping Fred's flat in a reasonable state of hygiene was important as he was unable to achieve this by himself and was in danger of losing the flat if it was not kept up to standard. This also provided the opportunity for Fred and the charge nurse to chat while carrying out the task.
- The clinical psychologist would spend half an hour a week chatting with Fred, choosing a time when he was behaving appropriately.
- All members of the staff team would make an effort to talk to Fred when he was behaving appropriately.

The next step was to decide how to monitor Fred's behaviour, as the day unit was a large one, with many places where members of his own staff team might not be able to observe his behaviour. It was agreed that it was possible to monitor his behaviour:

- in the canteen;
- on each of the three team bases;
- in the main reception area.

The day was then divided into four monitoring periods:

- breakfast
- 9 a.m.–12 noon
- lunch
- 2–5 p.m.

Fred could earn one point at the end of each time period if he had not carried out any unacceptable behaviours.

'Shall I sew some on for you?'
'No. If you give me buttons and thread, I'll do it.'
And he did. He did it well, and was very proud of the results.

4.2.4 DIRECT TREATMENT OF SYMPTOMS

After enthusiasm for token economy programmes declined, there followed a period in which little interest was shown by cognitive–behaviour therapists in the symptoms of schizophrenia, the most frequent diagnosis of people looked after by rehabilitation and long-term care services. Bellack (1986) argued that this lack of interest was based on four misconceptions:

- that schizophrenia does not exist;
- that it is a biological disorder, so there is no role for behaviour therapy;
- that it is best treated by medication;
- that it is too severe for behaviour therapy.

More recently, interest in the symptoms of people with severe mental illness has increased, and there is a growing body of research about cognitive–behavioural interventions for this group of people (Birchwood and Tarrier, 1992; Birchwood and Shepherd, 1992) which, although in its infancy, has produced some encouraging results. Some examples of such interventions will be discussed below.

(a) Attempts to modify auditory hallucinations

Early attempts to modify hallucinations, based on social learning theories and using such methods as social reinforcement and time-out (Bulow, Oei and Pinkey, 1979), punishment, self-instructions and thought stopping (Alford, Fleece and Rothblum, 1982; Bentall, Higson and Lowe, 1987), did not prove very successful. The approaches sometimes succeeded in changing patients' verbalizations about their voices, but little change was affected in the symptoms themselves (Marzillier and Birchwood, 1981).

More recently, three kinds of intervention based on cognitive–behavioural techniques have attempted to modify auditory hallucinations. Such techniques tend to be used when patients have not responded well to medication.

The use of ear plugs.   Done, Frith and Owens (1986), for example, found that wearing a cotton wool ear plug in the dominant ear reduced the frequency and volume of auditory hallucinations. The effect is thought to be due to a state being created which is dissonant with

At the end of breakfast and lunch, a nominated member of staff who had supervised the meal phoned the team base and reported on Fred's behaviour. At the end of the morning and afternoon periods Fred's key worker phoned the monitoring areas to ask for information about his behaviour. Once the information had been obtained, a chart was filled in, preferably with Fred present so that he would be praised for behaving appropriately or told why he had not earned the point. When Fred had earned four points he was able to have lunch in the canteen and was given a chit signed by a member of staff authorizing the canteen staff to give him a meal. The handing over of the chit also provided an opportunity for Fred to be praised.

Once the programme had been written, it was explained to Fred. Beyond the expectation of everyone, Fred consistently earned his points from the day the programme was started. His behaviour only deteriorated when staff became lax about carrying it out. It is of course important that once a programme has been set up, it must be maintained, and may need to be maintained for months or years. It is not uncommon for staff to complain that a patient is behaving badly again, and on investigation for it to be found that they have become lax about monitoring and rewarding the patient. How many employees would continue to go to work if they stopped being paid? It is not surprising that patients' behaviour deteriorates if a programme lapses. When setting up a behaviour management programme it is therefore important that the programme is:

- clearly written so that everyone can understand it;
- manageable by the staff on a long-term basis.

Particularly in non-hospital settings, with untrained staff, help may be sought in managing difficult behaviour, but the staff are reluctant to carry out a structured behaviour programme because it is so different from the way they are used to working. They sometimes feel that using a system of rewards is bribery. However, this reservation can usually be overcome by explaining that all of us, in our everyday lives, continue to do things that are rewarded and stop doing things that are not. Staff are usually more willing to try out a programme which they have designed with the clinical psychologist, so that they can be sure that the nature of the problems has been understood and that the programme agreed is manageable for them. It is also important to be available to answer any queries in the first few days of the programme's implementation and to review it after a few weeks so that it can be altered if it is not working.

4.2.3 SKILLS TRAINING

As has already been discussed in Chapter 2, the development of 'the physical, intellectual and emotional skills needed to live, learn, and work in the community' (Anthony, 1977) has been seen as central to the process of rehabilitation, particularly in the United States. The training of skills has focused on social and interpersonal skills (Appelo et al., 1992), problem-solving skills (Liberman et al., 1986), daily living skills (Wallace et al., 1992; Wallace, 1986) and vocational skills (Jacobs et al., 1992). As has already been discussed, a skills model of rehabilitation is not a sufficient model in itself. Nevertheless, the training of specific skills, or the maintenance of skills, may form part of an individual's care. In this instance, it is important to remember certain guidelines, and limitations.

(a) Be specific

Skills should be taught, as far as possible, in the environment in which they are to be used (Anthony, Cohen and Cohen, 1984). For example, if the aim is for the person to cook for him or herself at home, then teach the person in his or her own home. Where this is not possible, the training environment should simulate, as far as possible, the situation in which the patient is likely to be practising the skill. Many wards and hostels make the mistake of thinking that teaching a patient to cook meals for the six or more people living together in a hostel or on a ward will be sufficient training for catering for him or herself when living alone in a bedsit. Skills do not generalize well from one situation to another (Scott, Himadi and Keane, 1984; Appelo et al., 1992; Anthony, Cohen and Cohen, 1984). Anthony and co-workers (1984) suggest that, where an individual cannot be taught in the environment in which the skill is to be used, then 'generalization must be programmed' by teaching the skill in a variety of situations, teaching variations of response in the same situations, teaching self-evaluation and self-reward, and teaching the rules or principles which underlie the skill.

(b) Be systematic

Skills should be broken down into small, manageable steps (Wallace et al., 1992) which can be built up gradually.

(c) Don't make assumptions

It should not be assumed that an individual impaired in one skill will be globally impaired in all skills. Perkins and Dilks (1992) suggest

that developmental models are often used, either implicitly or explicitly, when patients are severely disabled. It is assumed, for example, that some skills are a prerequisite to other skills and so, for example, 'if a person cannot dress themselves properly, or behave appropriately at meal times then they cannot work or have political views or opinions' (Perkins and Dilks, 1992). Whereas a developmental model may be appropriate with children, it is not helpful in understanding the difficulties of people who are severely disabled by their mental illness.

> Severely socially disabled people, like severely physically disabled people, are multiply, but not universally, disabled. Each has an individual pattern of strengths and difficulties that do not follow a predetermined hierarchy or 'ladder' approach to rehabilitation: the person who is unable to wash, cook and budget their money unaided may well be able to paint, or to work in open employment. Adherence to a developmental perspective serves both to encourage infantilization and to neglect those areas of competency that the person has. The challenge is to optimise the person's strengths and abilities, whatever these might be, and to minimise the dismissive consequences of difficult behaviours and disabilities. (Perkins and Dilks, 1992).

The following examples illustrate the sorts of mistake staff make in assuming that patients are globally, rather than multiply, impaired.

- Andy lived on a hostel-ward and was unable to carry out most activities of daily living without a large amount of help. He spent most of the days scavenging for discarded food or drinks, despite being well fed at the hostel. His key nurses noticed that he needed a new pair of shoes and debated how to find out his size, as he would not co-operate with going around shops and trying shoes on. Eventually they settled on drawing round his foot on piece of paper.   While in the process of trying to do this another member of staff came along.
  'What are you doing?'
  'Trying to find out what size shoes Andy takes.'
  'Why don't you ask him? What size shoes do you take, A
  'Sevens.'
- Ralph had poor self-care, did not cook for himself or clean and did little all day despite the attempts of staff to occupied. For several days he had been going around with most of the buttons missing, until someone deci a solution.
  'It's a shame about your missing buttons, Ralph.'
  'Yes, it's cold.'

the subjective localization of the voices. The patient experiences the voices as coming from, for example, the right side and so 'believes' that they cannot be heard so clearly when there is a plug in the right ear.

The use of headphone music.   For example, Hustig *et al.* (1990) and Morley (1987). It has been found that for some people music, radio or white noise played on a personal stereo with headphones can reduce the volume or intrusion of auditory hallucinations. The type of noise that is effective appears to be idiosyncratic, some people preferring loud music such as heavy metal, which one might expect to be over-stimulating, and others preferring something quiet or soothing. However, this intervention has not been effective for all people and for some it has made the symptoms worse, perhaps by acting as an additional stressor.

Enhancing people's own coping strategies.   Tarrier *et al.* (1990), for example, have developed coping strategy enhancement (CSE) as a way of helping people to cope with their auditory hallucinations. They suggest that everyone attempts to cope with their own symptoms one way or another and so one might capitalize on, and enhance, these attempts. There are eight stages to CSE intervention:

1. explaining the rationale to the patient;
2. eliciting and defining the symptoms;
3. carrying out a behavioural analysis of the symptoms, such as analysing their frequency, duration and severity, their antecedents, the behaviour of the patient and the consequences of that behaviour;
4. clarifying the patient's coping strategies as appropriate or inappropriate – for example, long-term social withdrawal is inappropriate, temporary social disengagement appropriate;
5. teaching the patient to monitor the symptoms;
6. targeting the symptoms for intervention;
7. identifying potential coping strategies;
8. practising carrying out the coping strategies when the symptoms occur.

Examples of behavioural strategies used for coping with hallucinations are attending to external stimuli, thought stopping and engaging in alternative behaviour. Although CSE has had some limited success, Tarrier *et al.* (1990) point out that the coping strategies sometimes do not generalize to use outside the practice sessions, and suggest that this may be because patients believe the voices they hear are real, rather than coming from inside their heads, and so do not think it appropriate to engage in the coping strategies or realize that they should be doing so at that point in time.

(b) Attempts to modify delusions

Recently, researchers and clinicians have begun to examine the thinking and reasoning styles associated with delusions (Bentall, 1992). It has been shown that deluded subjects 'jump to conclusions' when making decisions or inferences, and make less use of disconfirming information (Huq, Garety and Hemsley, 1988); and that subjects with persecutory delusions tend to attribute negative events to an external source (Bentall, 1992). These findings have led to the development of interventions which use cognitive techniques to manage delusions, for example the work of Chadwick and Lowe (1990). Their intervention has three stages.

1. Interviews are used to establish the belief which will be the target of intervention.
2. As much information as possible is gathered about the nature of the belief, including any evidence that has helped to establish and maintain the beliefs, and the patient is asked to rank each piece of evidence in order of importance to the belief system.
3. The patient is encouraged to view the belief as only one possible interpretation of the situation, and to consider alternatives. After discussing all the evidence for the belief, the belief itself is challenged.

Throughout the intervention, the stance taken by the therapist is non-confrontational, with an emphasis on making clear the way that beliefs can influence the interpretations made of situations and events. Such interventions are still in their infancy, awaiting the results of large scale studies.

While such approaches are increasing in popularity, Perkins and Dilks (1992) sound a note of caution, particularly when working with severely socially disabled people. Such people, who have often been in psychiatric services for many years, are likely to have had their distressing delusions met by three kinds of response because of the popular myth that one should never collude with delusions (Watts, Powell and Austin, 1973): the beliefs are ignored, for example the member of staff pretends that he or she did not hear the person talking about them; the person is diverted from talking about them; or the beliefs are challenged – the person is told that they are wrong. Perkins and Dilks (1992) suggest that 'to deny another's reality, to ignore and divert what may be very frightening experiences, serves to further isolate them and effectively prevents the formation of a good working relationship'. They suggest that the clinician should acknowledge the impact or emotional content of the person's experience, listening and sympathizing, or acknowledge that everyone's reality is different so that, while one can accept the other person's experiences as 'real' for them, it is not the way that others see things. This then leaves the way open for exploring the impact of the person's beliefs on his/her life and investigating ways of minimizing any negative effects they may have. The following case example illustrates this approach.

Matthew believed that his mental illness was the result of permanent damage to his nerves caused by too much sex in his youth, and 'burning the candle at both ends'. As a consequence he believed that his current level of functioning could not improve, that he had to eat well to feed his damaged nerves, and that he could not exercise, because of the damage. This resulted in him becoming obese. On many occasions, staff had told him that his beliefs were wrong, that this was not the cause of his problems and that he should be able to do more than he was doing. This had only served to confirm his belief that he had a special and severe kind of nerve damage which even the doctors did not understand and to make it even less likely that he would accept what staff said. Later, a new approach was taken with him. The emphasis was shifted toward accepting his interpretation of the situation, acknowledging how difficult that must make life for him, and helping him to find ways of coping despite his severe and permanent nerve damage. From then, his mood lifted, his self-esteem increased, he went daily and punctually to his sheltered work, and he moved from a hostel to an independent bedsit.

(c) Preventing or minimizing relapse

Work by Birchwood (1992) has suggested that cognitive–behavioural techniques aimed at enhancing coping strategies may help patients who are prone to frequent periods of relapse. The approach concentrates on identifying the unique characteristics of 'relapse signature' for a particular patient, which usually has two stages: dysphoria (including anxiety, restlessness, blunting of drives), followed by early psychotic symptoms (including suspiciousness, ideas of reference, misinterpretations). Intervention should consist of educating patients and their families about prodromes – the symptoms which herald relapse – and the early intervention possibilities which are available; helping the patient and the family to identify the individual's unique 'relapse signature' symptoms; teaching the patient to seek help from the psychiatric service and to carry out stress management techniques; and emphasizing mastery and control, rather than catastrophizing the experience. This is an interesting and potentially useful approach, but its effectiveness needs further investigation.

(d) Cognitive behavioural approaches to other disorders.

The interventions discussed above are recent innovations in the cognitive–behavioural treatment of people with schizophrenia. Although schizophrenia is a common diagnosis for people with long-term and severe mental health problems, it is by no means the only one. This patient group can, and does, suffer from a variety of disabling symptoms, such as obsessive–compulsive disorders, affective disorders, severe neurotic disorders, or combinations of these. Traditional cognitive–behavioural techniques can often be used to help patients cope with their symptoms, such as cognitive therapy for depression and systematic desensitization for a phobia.

However, such interventions, aimed at specific symptoms, must be carried out in the context of the individual's total care, and be consistent with the general philosophy of care adopted for that individual. This state of affairs is much more likely if the therapist is a member of the multidisciplinary team looking after that individual, rather than an outsider called in to carry out a single intervention. If the intervention is made out of context, then it is likely to become yet another failed treatment in the long history of the individual's psychiatric career. It is also important to remember that individuals are in rehabilitation and long-term care services because their symptoms are severe and long-term. Interventions aimed at specific symptoms will need to be slow, and long-term with an emphasis on coping rather than curing. Viewing the intervention in the context of the individual's total care will help the therapist not to inflate its importance, or to raise false expectations in the client.

4.3 COUNSELLING

4.3.1 DEFINITIONS OF COUNSELLING

'Being told what you already know by higher authority' (patient); 'constructive criticism' (manager); 'third-rate psychotherapy' (doctor); 'being told off by your boss' (nurse); 'helpful advice' (client); 'everybody does it' (psychotherapist). These random opinions, however apparently conflicting, suggest that counselling, in common with the multitude of psychotherapies, relies on time set aside for talking with a view to effecting change. In fact, counselling is often described in terms which either identify it implicitly as a form of psychotherapy (Stewart, 1985) or do so explicitly, as in the classification of psychotherapy levels by Cawley (1977):

1. outer level (support and counselling) which consists of unburdening of problems to a sympathetic listener, ventilation of feelings within a supportive relationship and discussing current problems with a non-judgemental helper;
2. intermediate level, which includes further clarification of problems and their origins within a deeper relationship, confrontation of defences and interpretation of unconscious motives and transference phenomena;
3. deeper level (exploration and analysis), which is based on remembering and reconstruction of the past, regression to less adult and less rational functioning and resolution of conflicts by experiencing and working through.

This useful grouping, however, does not sufficiently emphasize one of the main reasons for separating counselling from other psychotherapies; the term 'counselling', more often than not, signifies advice, which clearly distinguishes it from insight-oriented psychotherapy.

4.3.2 COUNSELLING IN REHABILITATION

Counselling is an essential rehabilitation tool (Ekdawi, 1981); in contrast, the deeper levels of psychotherapy are not considered to be appropriate in the treatment and rehabilitation of people with psychotic disorders, who are the main concern of rehabilitation services. Freud (1953), for instance, stated that persons with schizophrenia were unsuitable subjects for psychoanalytic enquiry because of their inability to form a transference neurosis. A number of sophisticated comparative studies, exemplified by Gunderson et al. (1984), failed to show that insight-oriented psychotherapy was superior to supportive psychotherapy or drug treatment in schizophrenia. They also concluded that supportive psychotherapy patients functioned more independently, spent less time in hospital and were more likely to be employed than those who received the more traditional forms of psychotherapy.

These studies, moreover, were not concerned with people with long-term disabling illnesses, where deeper level psychotherapies could either be highly stressful, leading to an increase in the severity of positive symptoms, or inappropriate, in cases where cognitive impairments make it difficult to cope with abstract ideas.

4.3.3 ELEMENTS OF REHABILITATION COUNSELLING

(a) Principles

Rehabilitation counselling, together with other rehabilitation interventions, aims at reducing idiosyncratic, maladaptive reactions to environmental events, developing awareness into signs of impending symptom relapse (Carpenter, 1984) and strengthening coping abilities. As a first step, it is important to consider and to have some understanding of the person's attitudes and reactions to his disabilities – as a patient's father put it, 'you have to listen to his being'. These reactions could fall within two contrasting frameworks: a succumbing framework which concentrates on the difficulties and heartbreak of being a victim of illness and which emphasizes what the person cannot do, and a coping framework which is constructive and optimistic, concentrating on abilities and active community participation (Wright, 1984). These reactions have powerful influences on the course and outcome of rehabilitation (Wing, 1966) and it is therefore necessary for the counsellor to be aware of them when problems are being discussed.

The next step is to clarify and define the problems, which are often presented in a poorly defined, ambiguous way. This is followed by considering realistic solutions and choosing the most appropriate ones. It is important that these steps are based on an understanding of the patient's impairments and on an appreciation of the benefits and risks of psychological interventions.

(b) Form

Rehabilitation counselling may take the form of a limited number of sessions specifically aimed at a particular issue, such as giving advice on welfare benefits or imparting information on newly prescribed medication. In general, however, it is provided within the matrix of an established long-term supportive relationship, and here, continuity is vital; as one relative said, 'chronic patients need chronic staff'. It should always be remembered, at the same time, that deeper intimacy can be threatening and that, therefore, counselling sessions should not be too frequent.

(c) Content

Bachrach (1982) observed that the traditional forms of insight-oriented psychotherapy have limited relevance to the needs of most psychiatrically disabled people; she thought it important, in this context, that the meaning of insight should be redefined so that it applied to 'the here and now' and that counselling should be reality-based, with the focus on such matters as the effects of stress, the role and limitations of medication in controlling stress and the need to understand and, if possible, to avoid anxiety-provoking situations.

Lamb (1982) also commented on the great difficulty which people with long-term schizophrenic illnesses have in handling the closeness of intensive psychotherapy; he advocated a counselling structure based on a problem-solving approach, which has similarities to the model of rehabilitation counselling later propounded by Stewart (1985). Within such structure, ambiguity and long silences should be avoided during the sessions; psychotic talk and loss of control in expressing emotions, such as anger, should be discouraged. The accent should be on strengthening ego controls by encouraging reality thinking, by setting limits to behaviour and by giving directional advice simply and clearly. The main objectives should be to enhance the individual's capacity to attain mastery over internal and external demands and to expand the well part, rather than to remove or cure pathology. These themes are directly related to the concept of social disablement, whose fundamental standpoint is the person's relationship with the social environment.

Turning to some specific issues, there is evidence that counselling is more effective when it is clearly linked to a current personal problem. For example, a woman who was distressed at work because of her suspicion that her colleagues' chance remarks had a hidden meaning was receptive to the suggestion that her 'over-sensitivity' was related to her illness and she was therefore better able to cope with her persecutory feelings. On the other hand, more generalized information on illness, though occasionally of value, may be perceived as irrelevant or inappropriate (Pilsecker, 1981).

Coping with 'internal' abnormal experiences is a central issue. In a study of 50 patients with a diagnosis of schizophrenia, Dittman (1990) found that the majority had some understanding of their illness and that they tried to cope with their psychotic experiences in individually different ways. Methods of coping with symptoms and self-management are usually developed on a trial and error basis, but they do not always work. Of the patients surveyed by Tarrier (1987), 30% reported that their strategies of coping with symptoms were ineffective; however, multiple strategies can be built on, taught and systematically practised (Tarrier *et al.*, 1990).

Learning to cope with external stresses can be enhanced by counselling. The whole range of life events, as well as long-term environmental difficulties, such as poor family relationships, have been known to contribute to symptom exacerbation and impaired social functioning. Many people with psychiatric disability acquire some appreciation of the links between these factors, often after prolonged experience and suffering (Wing, 1983). The process of appreciation, which is the first step towards coping, can be facilitated by counselling.

(d) Provisions

Given that counselling is an essential ingredient of the stock-in-trade of rehabilitation professionals, it follows that they should be trained in its principles and application. Difficulties in counselling which are imposed by severe disabilities and fluctuating insight can, to some extent, be mitigated by forming a long-term relationship; this relationship can be built up with the rehabilitation team so that counselling is provided by its members, using their differing skills and expertise. In choosing an appropriate counsellor, due regard should be given to personal attributes; the 'composed' counsellor, for example, tends to work well with anxious people, while one who is uncomfortable with aggression may find hostile individuals difficult (Gunderson, 1978).

There are advantages in group counselling in that it exploits the influences and experience of the individual's reference group. It also provides effective mutual support.

In planning individual and group counselling, it is essential to pay a great deal of attention to practical arrangements such as the location of the sessions, their timing, transport arrangements, etc. (Ekdawi, 1981; Wilson, 1986).

4.3.4 COUNSELLING RELATIVES

There is a wealth of literature which indicates that supportive counselling of relatives is a highly effective rehabilitation intervention. Various models have been successfully used (Falloon *et al.*, 1982; Kuipers *et al.*, 1989; Smith and Birchwood, 1990); their common ground is that relatives are a valuable resource in the management of people with psychiatric disability. Such family interventions have been shown to result in favourable changes in attitudes, thus maximizing the families' effectiveness in working in partnership with the professionals, and in ultimately reducing morbidity.

The origins of both positive and negative family attitudes and reactions to their disabled member, to the consequences of the illness and to the treatment are highly complex; they are also extremely difficult to fit into simple theoretical frameworks. Goldstein (1987), for instance, pointed out that high levels of expressed emotion could relate to coping mechanisms used by relatives to handle massive difficulties and that they are not necessarily the cause of the difficulties. Over 30 years' experience of relatives' counselling and support groups at Netherne Hospital, England, has made it evident to the rehabilitation staff that relatives need clear information and advice rather than therapy, so that they can cope effectively.

First and foremost, they need to know what it is that they have to cope with; 'it is not appropriate for relatives to play guessing games (about diagnosis) nor to rely on hearing remarks dropped accidentally by a nurse or on being told by another patient' (Weleminsky, 1991). They also require concrete advice on how to communicate with the patient, how to deal with difficult behaviour and disturbed talk without being too intrusive or 'over-protective', on the role of medication and on setting realistic expectations regarding work and socialisation (National Schizophrenia Fellowship, 1980). Guidance on practical matters, such as welfare benefits and on the correct channels for obtaining help in emergencies is often sought.

In every instance, counselling should be intelligible and explicit and it should be within the counsellor's competence and knowledge. In communicating with relatives, it is vital to avoid over-simplification as well as technical jargon; both can erect barriers and raise anxiety levels (Hatfield, 1986). Families harbour feelings of guilt, shame and embarrassment; the use of judgemental language which may suggest that relatives intentionally cause harm to the patients should be avoided. Hatfield also criticized professionals' tendency to stereotype families by placing them into either/or categories, for example, disturbed families, problem families and high EE families; such language, apart from being inaccurate, can be confusing, stigmatizing and offensive. To some extent, group counselling with families can reduce the risks of communication difficulties – there is safety in numbers. Group counselling also has the advantages of mutual support and the opportunity to learn from others who have had first hand experience; 'a family hit by the illness is like a kamikaze pilot – it is a one-off experience with disastrous consequences, and you need all the help you can get from others who have been through it,' said one relative.

The creation of a healthy partnership between relatives and professionals is dependent on mutual respect and on the recognition that each has valuable contributions to the care and rehabilitation of disabled people. This does not apply only to the care of individuals; a cohesive relatives' group has the potential of positive political influence, giving assistance and support in the planning, monitoring and improving the quality of service provision.

REFERENCES

Alford, G.S., Fleece, L. and Rothblum, E. (1982) Hallucinatory-delusional verbalisations: modification in a chronic schizophrenic with self-control and cognitive restructuring. *Behaviour Modification*, **6**, 421–435.

Allyon, T. and Azrin, N.H. (1968) *The Token Economy: a Motivational System for Therapy and Rehabilitation*, Appleton-Century-Crofts, New York.

Anthony, W.A. (1977) Psychological Rehabilitation: a concept in need of a method. *American Psychologist*, **Aug**, 658–662.

Anthony, W.A., Cohen, M.R. and Cohen, B.F. (1984) Psychiatric rehabilitation, in *The Chronic Mental Patient: Five Years Later*, (ed. J.A. Talbott), Grune & Stratton, Orlando, FL, Ch. 10.

Appelo, M.T., Woonings, F.M.J., Van Nieuwenhuizen, C.J. (1992) Specific skills and social competence in schizophrenia. *Acta Psychiatrica Scandinavica*, **85**, 419–422.

Attwood, N. and Beck, J. (1985) Service and patient predictors of continuation in clinical based treatment. *Hospital and Community Psychiatry*, **36**, 865–870.

Bachrach, L.L. (1982) Foreword, in *Treating the Long-term Mentally Ill*, (ed. R.H. Lamb), Jossey-Bass, San Francisco.

Barton, R. (1959) *Institutional Neurosis*, John Wright, Bristol.

Bateson, G. (1961) *Perceval's Narrative: a Patient's Account of his Psychosis 1830–1832*, Hogarth Press, London.

Bellack, A. (1986) Schizophrenia: behaviour therapy's forgotten child. *Behaviour Therapy*, **17**, 199–214.

Bentall, R. (1992) Reconstructing psychopathology. *Psychologist*, **5**, 61–66.

Bentall, R.P., Higson, P.S. and Lowe, C.F. (1987) Teaching self-instructions to chronic schizophrenic patients: efficacy and generalisation. *Behaviour Therapy*, **15**, 58–76.

Birchwood, M. (1992) Early intervention in schizophrenia: theoretical background and clinical strategies. *British Journal of Clinical Psychology*, **31**, 257–278.

Birchwood, M. and Shepherd, G. (1992) Controversies and growing points in cognitive-behavioural interventions for people with schizophrenia. *Behavioural Psychotherapy*, **20**, 305–342.

Birchwood, M. and Tarrier, N. (1992) *Innovations in the Psychological Management of Schizophrenia*. John Wiley & Sons: Chichester.

Birley, J.L.T. and Brown, G.W. (1970) Crises and life changes preceding the onset or relapse of acute schizophrenia: clinical aspects. *British Journal of Psychiatry*, **126**, 327–333.

Bulow, H., Oel, T.P.S. and Pinkey, B. (1979) Effects of contingent social reinforcement with delusional chronic schizophrenic men. *Psychological Reports*, **44**, 659–666.

Cawley, R.H. (1977) The teaching of psychotherapy. *Association of University Teachers of Psychiatry Newsletter*, **Jan**, 19–36.

Carpenter, W.T. (1964) Thoughts on the treatment of schizophrenia. *Schizophrenia Bulletin*, **12**, 527–539.

Chadwick, P. and Lowe, F. (1990) The measurement and modification of delusional beliefs. *Journal of Consulting Clinical Psychology*, **58**, 225–232.

Christison, G.W., Darrell, G.K. and Wyatt, R.J. (1991) When symptoms persist: choosing among alternative somatic treatments for schizophrenia. *Schizophrenia Bulletin*, **17**, 217–245.

Conning, A.M. and Brownlow, J.M. (1992) Determining suitability of placement for long-stay psychiatric inpatients. *Hospital and Community Psychiatry*, **43**(7), 709–712.

Coppen, A. and Abou-Saleh, M.T. (1988) Lithium therapy: from clinical trials to practical management. *Acta Psychiatrica Scandinavica*, **28**, 754–762.

Crammer, J. and Heine, B. (1991) *The Use of Drugs in Psychiatry*, Gaskell, London.

Davis, H. and Fallowfield, L. (1991) *Counselling and Communication in Health Care*, John Wiley & Sons, Chichester.

Dittman, J. (1990) Disease consciousness and coping strategies of patients with schizophrenic psychosis. *Acta Psychiatrica Scandinavica*, **82**, 318–322.

Donaldson, S.R., Gelenberg, A.J. and Baldessarini, R.J. (1983) The pharmacologic treatment of schizophrenia: a progress report. *Schizophrenia Bulletin*, **9**, 504–527.

Done, D.J., Frith, C.D. and Owens, D.C. (1986) Reducing persistent auditory hallucinations by wearing an ear-plug. *British Journal of Clinical Psychology*, **25**, 151–152.

Ekdawi, M.Y. (1981) Counselling in rehabilitation, in *Handbook of Psychiatric Rehabilitation Practice*, (eds J.K. Wing and B. Morris), Oxford University Press, Oxford.

Falloon, I.R.H., Boyd, J.L., McGill, C.W. *et al.* (1982) Family management in the prevention of exacerbations of schizophrenia – a controlled study. *New England Journal of Medicine*, **306**, 1437–1440.

Freud, S. (1953) *Neuropsychoses of Defence*, Hogarth Press, London.

Goffman, I. (1961) *Asylums: Essays on the Social Situation of Mental Patients and Other Inmates*, Penguin Books, Harmondsworth, Middlesex.

Goldstein, M.J. (1987) Psychological issues. *Schizophrenia Bulletin*, **13**, 157–171.

Gripp, R.F. and Magaro, P.A. (1974) The Token Economy Program in the psychiatric hospital: a review and analysis. *Behaviour Research and Therapy*, **12**, 205–228.

Gunderson, J.G. (1978) Patient–therapist matching: a research evaluation. *American Journal of Psychiatry*, **135**, 1193–1197.

Gunderson, J.G., Frank, A.F., Katz, H.M. *et al.* (1984) Effects of psychotherapy in schizophrenia: II. Comparative outcome of two forms of treatment. *Schizophrenia Bulletin*, **10**, 564–598.

Hall, J., Baker, R.D. and Hutchinson, K. (1977) A controlled evaluation of token economy procedures with chronic psychiatric patients. *Behaviour Research and Therapy*, **15**, 261–283.

Hatfield, A.B. (1986) Semantic barriers to family and professional collaboration. *Schizophrenia Bulletin*, **12**, 325–333.

Higgins, D.L., Galavotti, C., O'Reilly, K.R. *et al.* (1988) Evidence for the effects of HIV antibody counselling and testing on risk behaviours. *Journal of the American Medical Association*, **266**, 2419–2429.

Hill, B.A. (1988) Factors influencing satisfaction and successful placement in hostels for people with a long-term psychiatric disability. University of London. MSc thesis.

Hogarty, G.E. (1984) Depot neuroleptics. The relevance of psychosocial factors. *Journal of Clinical Psychiatry*, **45**, 36–42.

Holloway, F. (1988) Prescribing for the long-term mentally ill. A study of treatment practices. *British Journal of Psychiatry*, **152**, 511–515.

Huq, S.F., Garety, P. and Hemsley, D. (1988) Probabilistic judgements in deluded and non-deluded subjects. *Quarterly Journal of Experimental Psychology*, **40A**, 801–802.

Hustig, H.H., Tran, D.B., Hafner, R.J. and Miller, R.J. (1990) The effect of headphone music on persistent auditory hallucinations. *Behavioural Psychotherapy*, **18**(4), 273–282.

Jacobs, H.E., Wissusik, D., Collier, R. *et al.* (1992) Correlations between psychiatric disabilities and vocational outcome. *Hospital and Community Psychiatry*, **43**(4), 365–369.

Johnson, D.A.W., Pasterski, G., Ludlow, J.M. *et al.* (1983) The discontinuance of maintenance neuroleptic therapy in chronic schizophrenic patients: drugs and social consequences. *Acta Psychiatrica Scandinavica*, **67**, 339–352.

Johnson, D. (1990) Long-term drug treatment of psychosis: observations on some current issues. *International Review of Psychiatry*, **2**, 341–353.

Johnstone, E.C., Crow, T.J. and Firth, C.D. (1988) The Northwick Park 'functional' psychosis study: diagnosis and treatment response. *Lancet*, **ii**, 119–124.

Kazdin, A.E. (1978) *The Token Economy*, Plenum Press, New York.

Kelly, J.A. and St Lawrence, J.S. (1990) The impact of community based groups to help people to reduce HIV risk behaviours. *AIDS Care*, **2**, 25–26.

Kuipers, L., MacCarthy, B., Hurry, J. and Harper, R. (1989) Counselling the relatives of the long-term mentally ill: II. A low-cost supportive model. *British Journal of Psychiatry*, **154**, 775–782.

Lamb, H.R. (1982) *Treating the Long-term Mentally Ill*, Jossey-Bass, San Francisco.

Leff, J.P. and Wing, J.K. (1971) Trial of maintenance therapy in schizophrenia. *British Medical Journal*, **3**, 559–604.

Leff, J.P. and Vaughan, C. (1980) The interaction of life events and relatives' expressed emotion in schizophrenia and depressive neurosis. *British Journal of Psychiatry*, **136**, 146–153.

Liberman, R.P. and Evans, K.C. (1985) Behavioural rehabilitation for chronic mental patients. *Journal of Clinical Psychopharmacology*, **5**, 85–145.

Liberman, R.P., Mueser, K.T., Wallace, C.J. *et al.* (1986) Training skills in the psychiatrically disabled: learning coping and competence. *Schizophrenia Bulletin*, **12**(4), 631–647.

Marzillier, J.S. and Birchwood, M. (1981) Behaviour therapy of schizophrenic disorders, in *Future Perspectives in Behaviour Therapy*, (eds L. Michelson, M. Hessen and A. Ballack), Plenum Press, New York.

May, P.R.A. (1976) When, what and why? Psychopharmacotherapy and other treatments in schizophrenia. *Comprehensive Psychiatry*, **17**, 683–693.

Miller, K., Donegan, E., Curran, P. *et al.* (1990) Effects of counselling on knowledge about HIV-1 among transfusion recipients and their partners. *AIDS Care*, **2**, 155–162.

Morley, S. (1987) Modification of auditory hallucinations: Experimental studies of headphones and ear plugs. *Behavioural Psychotherapy*, **15**, 240–251.

National Schizophrenia Fellowship (1980) *Social Provision for Sufferers from Chronic Schizophrenia*, National Schizophrenia Fellowship, Surbiton.

Paul, G.L. and Lentz, R.J. (1977) *Psychosocial Treatment of Chronic Mental Patients: Milieu vs Social-Learning Programmes*, Harvard University Press, Cambridge, MA.

Perkins, R. and Dilks, S. (1992) Worlds apart: Working with severely socially disabled people. *Journal of Mental Health*, **1**, 3–17.

Pilsecker, C. (1981) On educating schizophrenics about schizophrenia. *Schizophrenia Bulletin*, **7**, 379–382.

Quitkin, F.M., Kane, J., Rifkin, A. *et al.* (1981) Prophylactic lithium carbonate with and without imipramine for bipolar 1 patients. *Archives of General Psychiatry*, **38**, 902–907.

Scott, R.R., Himadi, W. and Keane, T.M. (1984) A review of generalisation in social skills training: suggestions for future research. *Progress in Behaviour Modification*, **15**, 113–172.

Smith, J. and Birchwood, M. (1990) Relative and patients as partners in the management of schizophrenia – the development of a service model. *British Journal of Psychiatry*, **156**, 654–660.

Soni, S.D., Sampath, G., Shah, A. and Krska, J. (1992) Rationalising neuroleptic polypharmacy in chronic schizophrenics: effects of changes to a single depot preparation. *Acta Psychiatrica Scandinavica*, **85**, 354–359.

Stewart, W. (1985) *Counselling in Rehabilitation*, Croom Helm, London.

Tantum, D. (1992) The contribution of psychotherapy to rehabilitation. Netherne Hospital, Freudenberg Lecture, 14.5.92.

Tarrier, N. (1987) An investigation of residual psychotic symptoms in discharged schizophrenic patients. *British Journal of Clinical Psychology*, **26**, 141–143.

Tarrier, N., Harwood, S., Yusopoff, L., Beckett, R. and Baker, A. (1990) A coping strategy enhancement (CSE): a method of treating residual schizophrenic symptoms. *Behavioural Psychotherapy*, **18**(4), 283–294.

Van Putten, T. (1974) Why do schizophrenic patients refuse to take their drugs? *Archives of General Psychiatry*, **31**, 67–72.

Waismann, L.C. (1988) Needs and other motivational processes in long-term psychiatric patients in an era of community care. University of London, PhD thesis.

Wallace, C.J. (1986) Functional Assessment in Rehabilitation. *Schizophrenia Bulletin*, **12**(4), 604–630.

Wallace, C.J., Liberman, R.P., MacKain, S.J. *et al.* (1992) Effectiveness and replicability of modules for teaching social and instrumental skills to the severely mentally ill. *American Journal of Psychiatry*, **149**(5), 654–658.

Waters, M.A. and Northover, J. (1965) Rehabilitated long-stay schizophrenics in the community. *British Journal of Psychiatry*, **111**, 258–263.

Watts, F.N., Powell, G.E. and Austin, S.V. (1973) The modification of abnormal beliefs. *British Journal of Medical Psychology*, **46**, 359–363.

Weleminski, J. (1991) Schizophrenia and the family – the customers' view. *International Review of Psychiatry*, **3**, 119–124.

Wilson, J. (1986) *Self-help Groups: Getting Started – Keeping Going*. Longmans, Harlow, Essex.

Wing, J.K. (1966) Social and psychological changes in a rehabilitation unit. *Social Psychiatry*, **1**, 21–28.

Wing, J.K. and Brown, G.W. (1970) *Institutionalism and Schizophrenia*, Cambridge University Press, Cambridge.

Wing, J. (1983) Schizophrenia, in *Theory and Practice of Psychiatry Rehabilitation*,

(eds F.N. Watts and D.H. Bennett), John Wiley & Sons, Chichester.
Wright, B.A. (1984) Developing constructive views of life with a disability, in *Rehabilitation Psychology*, (ed. D.W. Krueger), Aspen Systems Corporation, Rockville, CT.

Sheltered Environments

5

5.1 WORK

Work is the rehabilitation tool which has endured the longest and which has brought about the most positive results (Schwartz, 1976), and yet its value is sometimes underrated by psychiatric services. In an elegant review, Rowland and Perkins (1988) commented that the word 'work' is variously used to refer to employment, to a role, to a task and to expended effort, all of which may relate to health and ill health. Work is not synonymous with employment; according to Hartley (1980), purposeful activity which structures time, which entails effort and discretion and which has social significance can be defined as work, even though its performance may not attract financial remuneration based on the market value – hence voluntary work, housework and schoolwork. It is in this wider context that work has been considered to be the cornerstone of hospital and community rehabilitation programmes (Morgan and Cheadle, 1981; Lamb, 1982).

The opinion is sometimes expressed that people with psychiatric disability should not be expected to work, especially in times of high unemployment, and that, instead, they should engage in leisure pursuits. This is despite compelling evidence that the jobless often show global deterioration of social functioning, with loss of reality sense and loss of time sense, so that they are unable to take advantage of the available extra time by putting it to use in leisure activities (Jahoda, Lazenfeld and Zeisel, 1972). This is due not only to the obvious psychological and financial sequelae of unemployment, but also to lack of the daily structure imposed by work activities. People with psychiatric disability are particularly vulnerable to the negative effects of this loss of structure, which adds to their often considerable difficulties in initiating and maintaining recreational activities (Collis and Ekdawi, 1984), and may be significantly associated with increased severity of their symptoms (Wing and Brown, 1970). It has therefore been argued that they should have the opportunity to function in structured social roles, such as those provided by work, and that when such opportunities are scarce, they should be deprived of them last, rather than first (Shepherd, 1984).

There is also another, related notion that psychiatrically disabled people should have long periods of rest and relaxation rather than be exposed to the stress and hassle of work. While there are no grounds to believe that work can cure psychiatric symptoms, lack of work has significant adverse effects on health and social functioning, and the evidence is that it is an essential component of rehabilitation since it enables the disabled person to adapt to social demands (Rapoport, 1960). Most disabled people are fully aware of the deleterious effects of lack of work, as shown by the priority they accord to work in quality of life studies (Lehman, Ward and Linn, 1982) as well as in service consumer surveys (Rowland and Perkins, 1988). It is therefore appropriate to consider the relationship between work and health in some detail.

5.1.1 THE EFFECTS OF UNEMPLOYMENT ON HEALTH

Ill health can be the cause as well as the result of unemployment. There are disadvantages which are commonly found in association with unemployment and which have adverse effects on health: poverty, poor housing and rejection by society. In a comprehensive review of the subject, Smith (1987) pointed out that these are long-term effects and that the longer the state of unemployment persists, the greater the danger of the jobless person becoming discouraged, with a gradual loss of the desire and, to some extent, the capacity for work, thus passing from the status of the unemployed to that of the unemployable. Concurrently, there is an increase in health problems, with a significant rise in the rates of consultations with general practitioners (Higgs, 1981). In addition, there is an increase in mortality rates, and it was estimated by Brenner (1979) that unemployment in England and Wales was associated with tens of thousands of premature deaths. More recently, the same author studied the relationship between unemployment and mortality rates in Sweden, where there is an extensive welfare system geared to ameliorating the effects of joblessness; he concluded that there was a very strong probability that recession causes illness, with unemployment being the crucial variable (Brenner, 1987).

The evidence of the effects of joblessness on mental health is clearer and even more convincing than that for its effects on physical health. Warr (1985) found that there was an increase in anxiety, depression and neurotic disorders and a decrease in self-esteem and confidence, and he related these to nine factors: financial difficulties, restricted behaviours and environments, loss of 'traction' (the structure which pulls a person along and enables him to do other things including recreational activities), reduced opportunity and ability to make decisions, loss of motivation to develop new skills, increase in threatening and humiliating experiences, anxiety about the future, reduced amount and quality of personal contacts and decline in social status.

Other studies have also demonstrated that there was an increase in the rates of attempted suicide and deliberate non-fatal self-harm (Platt and Kreitman, 1984) and an association between unemployment and increased suicide rates (Moser *et al.*, 1987).

The suffering experienced by the families of the jobless cannot be overestimated: there is good evidence that marital relationships and relationships with children become strained and that there is higher incidence of ill health within the family (Smith, 1987).

5.1.2 UNEMPLOYMENT AND PSYCHIATRIC DISABILITY

Disabilities due to long-term unemployment may precede or follow chronic psychiatric illness, and they often form part of the complex picture of social disablement. Although a proportion of people with psychiatric disability are capable of employment, their prospects of securing jobs tend to be low; when unemployment levels in an area exceed 6%, there is a corresponding drop in the chances of employment for women, older people, ethnic minorities and disabled people. The lowest group in the pecking order is that of people with psychiatric disability. It was noted by Anthony, Cohen and Danley (1988) that, despite the central role of work in rehabilitation, a person discharged from a psychiatric hospital has a greater chance of returning to hospital than of returning to work. This is not because people choose the soft option of being unemployed, preferring to receive state benefit; a British Manpower Services national survey (Smith, 1987) showed that only 8% of the unemployed were not looking for work, usually because of their age. The majority thought that unemployment was bad for them. However, there comes a point when the motivation to seek jobs cannot be sustained in the face of continued rejection, and when disillusionment with job-finding services sets in, together with resignation to the fact that jobs are scarce anyway (Daniel, 1974).

Although public opinion towards mental illness is more enlightened, stigma still persists and employers are still reluctant to hire people with psychiatric disability, even when this is quite mild. This stems from the commonly held belief that people with a psychiatric history are unreliable or, alternatively, aggressive and destructive. Unfortunately, this image may sometimes be reinforced by the negative attitudes of some health professionals. It has been observed, however, that in the work environments, workmates and supervisors anticipate and experience less problems and hold more positive views, in working with their disabled colleagues, than managers and directors who have less direct contact with them.

Legislation against discrimination in employment is not always effective. Quota systems to assist the employment of disabled people are well-established in most Western countries, and in Britain, for example, a commercial firm has to employ disabled people in the ratio of 3% out of a work force of 20 or more. It is a law which is extremely difficult to enforce; preference is also often given to employing people with physical rather than psychiatric disabilities and, in any case, large statutory organizations such as the Health Service are exempt from it.

State welfare benefit systems, designed to assist disabled people, may actually discourage them from working. The rules do not usually allow for a long enough trial period in a job before benefits are stopped, and if the disabled employee leaves the job, even if this is because of illness, it may take much effort and time to re-establish benefits payments. Sickness and disability benefits often operate on an all-or-none basis; they do not allow for the fact that a person may be sick but capable of some work, and they make it almost impossible for a disabled person to work part-time.

In conclusion there is substantial evidence that unemployment is responsible for increased morbidity and mortality, that its effects are particularly detrimental to mental health and that it is associated with increased psychiatric disability. Rather than mitigating these effects, social factors, public attitudes and legislation may actually aggravate them.

5.2 WORK REHABILITATION

The value of work as a vehicle of social stimulation was clearly demonstrated in an experiment by Wing and Freudenberg (1961); the social behaviour of severely disabled chronic schizophrenic patients in a hospital workshop decidedly improved under favourable supervision conditions. Although their ward social behaviour did not show corresponding positive changes, this was possibly due to the experiment's short duration (6 weeks). In a 4 year study, where work was an integral component of the rehabilitation programme of a similar group of patients, ward behaviour improved and there was significant reduction in their social withdrawal and socially embarrassing behaviour (Ekdawi, 1966). The classical study, spanning 8 years, in which the social environments of three large mental hospitals were compared, clearly showed that the clinical deterioration in chronic schizophrenic patients was significantly associated with lack of occupation (Wing and Brown, 1970). For severely disabled people, therefore, work has positive effects on their social behaviour and on their symptoms.

A work programme has also been shown to be highly effective in the rehabilitation of long-term disabled patients whose disabilities were less severe (Wing 1966); the programme did not only improve their task performance, it also fostered constructive social behaviours compatible with job tenure. Difficulties in achieving work adjustment are not solely due to atrophy of work skills following prolonged illness and hospitalization; they are also caused by personality problems and attitudes (Jones, 1956). A study of 212 disabled people passing through an industrial rehabilitation unit showed that the social influences of the unit, such as identification with a reference group where realistic confidence and willingness to master the effects of disability were valued, were crucial in effecting good outcome (Wing, 1966). Among the factors which determine employability of people with psychiatric disability, good social relationships and appropriate social behaviour were highly significant (Watts, 1978), hence the emphasis on developing them in work rehabilitation programmes.

Work rehabilitation must not be seen as only relevant to future employment, but also to the process of social integration. It has been shown that patients working in hospital workshops were able to build up friendships and to relate to each other and to their supervisors in a socially acceptable manner (Miles, 1971). The performance of a work role, even in the most sheltered settings, is both a means and a measure of social adjustment, and it is perceived as such by disabled people and by those in contact with them (Collis and Ekdawi, 1984).

5.2.1 PROVISIONS FOR WORK REHABILITATION

There are many models and patterns in the provisions of work rehabilitation systems. The type, number and organization of facilities depend on the needs of the populations served, the characteristics of the geographical area and the types of available work. There are, however, certain essential components.

- A dedicated, multidisciplinary rehabilitation team: since social disablement is an amalgam of clinical disorder and social difficulties, a combined professional approach is essential. The sharp split, occasionally found in some programmes, between medical and vocational rehabilitation services is counter-productive and may undermine the programme's effectiveness (Lang and Rio, 1989).

- A central facility for assessment, planning and implementing interventions and preparation for resettlement in appropriate work environments: it is preferable that this should be a community-based day unit, since the direct transition from the status of hospital inpatient to that of worker is too great (Wansbrough and Cooper, 1980).
- A co-ordinated chain of work provisions, from open employment opportunities to very sheltered environments.
- Support systems for the workers, the employers, the staff of the work facilities and the families.

5.2.2 SOME EXAMPLES OF WORK REHABILITATION PROVISIONS

(a) Day rehabilitation units

A community based day rehabilitation unit should be centrally sited in the area it serves and it should be easily accessible by public transport. It has been estimated that such a unit should have 25–30 places for a district population of 200 000 (Acharya *et al.*, 1982). A high multidisciplinary staffing level is required, with direct supervision of the work areas given by industrially trained personnel. The unit provides a framework for assessment, training in work and related social skills such as time-keeping, social interactions and perseverance, as well as individually targeted medical, social and psychological interventions. A realistic work environment, providing a variety of paid, realistic work tasks is essential. The main functions of the unit are those summarized by Lang and Rio (1988):

- rehabilitation diagnosis, by a process of repeated assessments;
- rehabilitation planning, with agreed decisions on the goals to be achieved;
- rehabilitation interventions which rely on enabling the disabled person to make choices, develop skills and practise work adjustment activities.

Other important interventions include relief of symptoms, stabilizing of long-term medication and training in other skills as appropriate to the individual's needs. The unit could also provide the base of the rehabilitation team, back-up clinical services for the community work units and a centre for the follow-up and support of the workers.

Although there is no time limit of stay, the expectation is that people will move on to other work settings, bearing in mind that the process of work rehabilitation is often slow.

(b) Open employment

About 15–40% of people with psychiatric disability are capable of maintaining competitive employment, and it is essential that this significant proportion should not be denied the opportunity. Their survival in employment depends on the employer accepting the employee and on the employee tolerating the job (Watts, 1983). In order to achieve this, the rehabilitation programme should include accurate assessment, opportunities to acquire the necessary adaptive skills, finding the right job, training in the skills of securing employment and providing support.

In a follow-up study of employed people disabled by schizophrenia, Floyd (1983) found that stresses in the work environment, rather than dismissal, were the major cause of loss of employment. He concluded that these stresses can be minimized if the work environment provided some scope for learning and for freedom to organize the work, working in a small group with a good social climate, being busy most of the time with more emphasis on the quality of work than on its amount and having good supervision and feedback on performance. In effect, a degree of 'shelter' in a supportive environment may well be required for some disabled people to maintain open employment.

(c) Sheltered employment

The assumption that open employment is the ultimate aim of work rehabilitation is unrealistic and can only result in disillusionment and frustration. When employment was plentiful in the 1960s and 1970s, a follow-up study of 367 carefully selected and intensively trained moderately disabled hospital patients showed that only one third could sustain open employment (Ekdawi, 1972).

Sheltered employment, as distinct from sheltered work, gives some disabled people the opportunity to earn their living within the conditions and disciplines of open employment while being afforded certain concessions. This can be organized in sheltered factories, such as the British Remploy factories, or in schemes where an individual or a group can work in ordinary commercial settings alongside the 'able-bodied' workforce. Such schemes, for example the Sheltered Placement Scheme in Britain, may provide a permanent niche for those unsuited to open employment or, occasionally, a period of further rehabilitation leading to open employment.

Results of such schemes have shown that some 'poor risk' groups can perform satisfactorily, and even beyond what was expected (Daniels, 1966). In addition, many of these schemes have advantages over sheltered factories: they do not involve large capital investments, they do not segregate disabled people and they provide a greater variety of work in diverse settings. Their disadvantages are that they require the full co-operation of different agencies, which may be difficult to achieve; they also rely on marketing individual workers to as many employers, and in Britain, for example, it takes three times as long to find such placements for people with mental health problems than for the physically disabled.

In all sheltered employment placements, allowances are made for below average productivity and wages are therefore subsidized; very few, however, are flexible enough to take into account either marked fluctuations in performance or long periods of absence due to illness.

The estimated need of eight sheltered employment places for a population of 200 000 (Ekdawi, 1972) was made in a decade of full employment and was therefore too conservative.

(d) Training for employment

The plethora of statutory training schemes for the long-term unemployed can sometimes be exploited for the rehabilitation of people with mild or moderate psychiatric disability. They have the advantages of providing stimulating learning experiences in an enthusiastic atmosphere. Their fast pace and high levels of social stimulation, however, may precipitate symptom relapse (Wing, Bennett and Denham, 1964). Specially developed training schemes for people with psychiatric disability, exemplified by the Industrial Therapy Organizations pioneered by Early (1960) have achieved results in terms of employment resettlement; the most enduring, however, have been those which evolved according to changes in local employment conditions and which were linked with sheltered work facilities for those people who could not be placed in open employment.

(e) Sheltered workshops

In his study of industrial rehabilitation, Wing (1966) asked a most pertinent question: should severely disabled people be excluded from work rehabilitation since they are highly unlikely to progress to employment? The long history of industrial work provisions for long-term mental hospital patients, its rationale, functions and results were reviewed by Morgan (1983). The image of hospital industrial therapy workshops has undergone many changes over the decades; their critics thought that they encouraged unrealistic expectations for future employment and that the repetitive and low-paid work increased the risks of institutionalism. Such criticisms were not supported by research results (Freudenberg, 1960; Miles, 1971; Acharya *et al.*, 1982);

industrial workshops are still a valuable resource for severely disabled people who need supervision, support, social contacts and friendships, and a daily occupational structure in sheltered conditions. The closure of large mental hospitals has highlighted the need for similar provisions in the community, where the alternative is often doing nothing or aimlessly roaming the streets. The answer to Wing's question, therefore, must be that the most disabled have also great need for work rehabilitation.

Community workshops should preferably be sited within industrial areas, but they should have easy access to back-up clinical services. The number of workers in each workshop should be 20–30; the type and number of supervisory staff should reflect the workers' level of disability; severely disabled people may require high staffing levels and on-site clinical input, for example, from an occupational therapist.

Some community workshops are managed by, or firmly linked to health or social services; others, as has been the tradition in some European countries, operate independently of statutory services (Chatel and Joe, 1975). Good sheltered workshops should satisfy Warr's nine environmental attributes: opportunities for control, opportunities for skill use, externally generated goals, variety, environmental clarity, availability of money, physical security and valued social position (Warr, 1987). Many community workshops have expanded in the direction of manufacturing a variety of products (Grove, 1989) and of providing services (Mills, 1991). They evidently satisfy the users, as shown by the low levels of absenteeism (Ekdawi, 1989).

(f) Co-ordination of work rehabilitation

A chain of work rehabilitation services requires a high degree of co-ordination of the variety of organizations involved. Statutory employment agencies generally appoint special officers, whose knowledge of local commerce and industry equips them to represent the interests of disabled people, in liaison with the various agencies concerned. In Britain, this has traditionally been the role of the Disablement employment adviser (DEA), and while some DEAs have worked effectively with psychiatric rehabilitation teams, others have contributed very little in this field because of their inadequate training, their large workloads and their reluctance to tackle the problems of people with a history of psychiatric illness. For these reasons, some rehabilitation services have developed posts of employment co-ordinators, working within their teams. Their functions include negotiating and facilitating work placements in a variety of settings, supporting people working in open and sheltered employment, maintaining regular contact with employers and work facilities and acting as a port of call when problems arise (Gloag, 1985).

(g) Support

No work rehabilitation system can survive for long without a network of support. Much can be learnt from a study of people with psychiatric disability in open employment (Wansbrough and Cooper, 1980); the findings apply equally well to other work settings, including the most sheltered. There was no single case of the 'assembly line' causing relapse of symptoms or absence from work; difficulties at work were caused by social and family problems and by relapses following life events or discontinuance of medication. It is in those areas that most support is needed.

- Supporting working people can be organized in a number of ways; apart from routine outpatient appointments and home visits, it is essential to respond quickly to requests for help. Support groups for disabled workers can be immensely valuable because of the shared common experiences (Ekdawi, 1981). Professional support at the workplace is appropriate in some circumstances, particularly during the settling-in period of a new placement; this, however, could also have the negative effects of singling out the worker and of attracting unnecessary complaints.
- The attitudes of employers and workshop staff to their disabled workers are influenced by the amount of support available to them; adequate, continuing support and the knowledge that someone can be readily contacted if problems arise are perceived as a lifeline. This might also favourably influence their attitude to offer a chance to newcomers (Wansbrough and Cooper, 1980). Conversely, lack of support was found to be the greatest source of anger amongst employers reluctant to hire disabled applicants (Scott, 1982), and managers of sheltered workshops who are not adequately supported are often disinclined to consider the kind of disabled person who needs their services most.
- Almost without exception, families prefer their disabled relative to be constructively occupied (Collis and Ekdawi, 1984). Many, however, need a good deal of support to enable them to understand the value of work rehabilitation and to adjust their expectations to a realistic level; some may encourage their relatives to seek and to engage in work which is too ambitious or too stressful, and others may discourage positive changes in case they 'rock the boat'. The majority need support in the painful process of coming to terms with facts of psychiatric disability and its effects on work including

loss of jobs, lowered earnings, absenteeism and fluctuating performance. The mutual support given in family groups is particularly helpful in this context.

5.2 ACCOMMODATION

The closure of the large psychiatric asylums, and the move towards 'care in the community' has meant that clinicians and service planners have spent a lot of time, and expended huge amounts of energy, in thinking about the accommodation of patients with long-term and severe mental health problems. Although other aspects of a patient's life and care, such as work, money and medication, may be as or more important to the individual, the fact remains that hospitals cannot close until the residents are found alternative homes, so minds have been particularly concentrated on this aspect of service planning. While many places have been slow to appreciate the need for, for example, day care, 'everyone appreciates the need to have somewhere to lay one's head'. (Rowland, Zeelan and Waismann, 1992).

When thinking about the accommodation needed by patients of a rehabilitation and long-term care service, a number of questions spring to mind.

- How many places are needed, and of what type?
- Who should provide the accommodation, and how will it be funded?
- What type of patient should live in what type of accommodation, and what makes for a successful placement?
- Should patients who are moving from one type of accommodation to another be prepared for the move and, if so, how?

Unfortunately, despite the need to develop accommodation for this client group, there is very little hard data with which to answer these questions fully, but what information there is will be examined.

5.2.1 HOW MANY PLACES ARE NEEDED AND OF WHAT TYPE?

Some districts have attempted to answer the question 'how many places?' with reference to national or regional norms. However, it is unlikely that sole reliance on norms will be anything other than misleading (Wing and Furlong, 1986) (see Chapter 3). Districts vary enormously in social and demographic factors, as well as other factors such as whether or not they have a mental hospital with large numbers of 'old long-stay' patients, the size of the 'never institutionalized' group of long-term patients and whether or not there are influential staff with special interests who have attracted a larger than average group of patients with particular needs, all of which will affect the accommodation needs of the local service (Garety, 1988).

Further hints about the size and range of accommodation that might be needed can be got from studies of who lives where in established services. For example, Conning and Rowland (1991) surveyed all the patients in touch with a service for people with long-term and severe psychiatric disabilities in South London, and found that 6.8% of patients were in inpatient beds, 16.8% lived in hostels with varying degrees of support, 45.5% lived with a family member (partner, parent, child or sibling), 29.3% lived alone and 2% lived in other accommodation such as with a friend. This profile of a well established service is somewhat different from the work of Bates and Walsh (1989), who looked at the accommodation of patients who had moved out of four rehabilitation wards in Nottingham. They found that 18.6% were in hospital, 2.3% were in prison, 34.9% lived in supported accommodation such as hostels, 16.3% lived with their families, and 27.9% lived alone. The differences between the two services in the percentage of people living with their families, or in hostel-type accommodation, is likely to reflect the difference in the length of time since, or whether, the patients had lived in a mental hospital.

Whereas studies such as these, once accumulated, will show the limits in the variability of proportions of patients in each type of accommodation, and the relationship between local social and demographic features and this variability, it would be unwise to plan the accommodation required by one service on the basis of where people live in another. The general principles underlying the estimation of population needs were discussed in Chapter 3.

In answer to the 'what type of accommodation?' question, services have come up with a bewildering array of facilities (Rowland, Zeelan and Waismann, 1992). Examples are therapeutic communities, halfway houses, group homes, staffed hostels, hostels for respite and crisis care, apartments with more or less support, and family fostering/supportive landlady placements. Accommodation varies in the nature and degree of help available, and in the number of other people who share the accommodation.

The emphasis in supported accommodation has been on group living (e.g. Weinman and Kleiner 1978; Rowland, Zeelan and Waismann, 1992; Apte, 1968; Dickey et al., 1986; Mowbray, Greenfield and Freddolino, 1992), particularly staffed hostels and group homes, perhaps because this is thought to prevent loneliness (Conning and Rowland, 1991) and because, in the form of an unstaffed, or minimally staffed group home, it is cheap (Rowland, Zeelan and Waismann, 1992). A few studies have examined residents' attitudes towards their group living arrangements, and whether or not they do prevent loneliness. Many people who live in hostels would prefer to live alone (Lehman, Ward and Linn, 1982; Kay and Legg, 1988; Nordentoft, Knudsen and Schulsinger, 1992) and are dissatisfied with their accommodation (Hill, 1988). Hostels do not foster close friendships between residents (Pritlove, 1983; Hill, 1988) and for some individuals the socially stimulating environment created by group living produces florid psychotic symptoms (Falloon and Marshall, 1983).

While our knowledge about the types of accommodation needed is so poor, the best solution is to provide a range of accommodation, shifting the emphasis from group living to single or couple units, perhaps with several units in one block providing the opportunity for socializing if required. It is now being realized that a high degree of staff support can be provided to people living in single accommodation: 'highly staffed' does not have to mean 'group living'. If the degree of staffing is not dependent on the physical construction of the building, then it becomes easier to use staff flexibly, giving more input when it is needed and withdrawing when it is not.

5.2.2 WHO SHOULD PROVIDE THE ACCOMMODATION AND HOW SHOULD IT BE FUNDED?

Some of the difficulties in funding residential places of people with long-term mental health problems, and the effects of legislation upon funding, are illustrated by developments in Britain. In 1975 the British Government White Paper *Better Services for the Mentally Ill* suggested that Social Services departments should provide four to six places per 100 000 of the population in short-stay hostels, 15–24 places per 100 000 in long-stay hostels, plus a range of accommodation without resident staff, such as group homes, flats and boarding-out schemes (Pritlove, 1983; Garety, 1988). This White Paper set targets for provision, stating that in England there should be 47 000 inpatient beds for the mentally ill, a decrease from the 104 400 places in 1975; there should be 11 500 residential places for the mentally ill in England, provided by local authorities, the private sector and the voluntary sector, an increase from 3500 places provided in 1974 (Rowland, 1990). In other words, 56,500 inpatient beds were to be replaced by an increase of only 8000 residential places.

The Government's aim was to change the overall balance of care from an almost total reliance on residential care to two-thirds residential and one-third supporting people in their own homes. By 1984, the funding of residential care places was as follows: Hospital inpatients 70 000 (92.5%), local government homes 2400 places (3%), private and voluntary homes 3300 places (5.5%) of which 1400 (2%) were funded by local government and 1900 (2.5%) by state benefits (Rowland, 1990), so there was still a long way to go to achieve the Government targets.

During the 1980s there was growing disquiet about the way the move towards care in the community was being implemented and particularly about its appropriateness for people with long-term and severe psychiatric disabilities (Rowland, 1990). Many people claimed that there was a failure to provide adequate accommodation for people who used to live in psychiatric institutions (e.g. Patrick, Higgit and Holloway, 1989; Garety, 1988), resulting in a growing number of mentally ill people being homeless (Priest, 1970, 1971; Lodge Patch, 1971; House of Commons Social Services Committee, 1985; Marshall, 1989: Abdul-Hamid and McCarthy, 1989; Nordentoft, Knudsen and Schulsinger, 1992).

Perhaps in response to this growing disquiet, in 1986 Sir Roy Griffiths was asked to undertake an overview of community care policy, and in particular 'to review the way in which public funds are used to support community care policy' and to advise on 'the options for actions that would improve the use of these funds as a contribution to more effective community care' (Griffiths, 1988). Many of his recommendations have been adopted in the National Health Service and Community Care Act (Department of Health, 1990). In particular, the Act makes the distinction between health/medical care, which remains the responsibility of the National Health Service, and social care, which becomes the responsibility of Social Services. This effectively shifts the responsibility for residential care (other than inpatient beds for medical care) into the hands of Social Services, although Social Services must consult with the Housing Authorities, voluntary Housing Associations and private organizations providing housing, as it is expected that the private sector and the voluntary sector will provide a growing proportion of housing for people with long-term and severe mental health problems.

The Act also aims to enable people to live in their own homes by promoting the development of domiciliary, day and respite services. However, it is likely that the changes to the financial arrangements made by the Act, implemented in April 1993, will hamper the role which the voluntary sector can play in providing accommodation. Prior to the implementation of the Act, people placed in hostels, group homes and so on had their accommodation financed by state benefits, from the Social Security budget. This budget was not cash-limited and so funding was as good as guaranteed for anyone already placed in residential care. After implementation, an amount of money was transferred from the Social Security budget to the local authority budget. This is a cash-limited budget and the transferred money is not ring-fenced for the mentally ill, and so can potentially be spent on whatever group the local authority considers a priority. As a consequence it may not be available to fund accommodation for people with long-term and severe mental health problems.

Prior to the implementation of the Act, accommodation for this client group was provided by a number of different agencies: the National Health Service, local authority Social Services, local authority housing departments, voluntary organizations and private organizations, not to mention families. What has been provided, and by whom, has varied enormously from district to district. For example, residential accommodation for people with long-term psychiatric disabilities in North Lincolnshire relies heavily on the private sector. In contrast, the majority of sheltered accommodation places for this client group in South Southwark are provided by the voluntary sector, although staff of the Health Authority play a major role in setting up and managing these voluntary housing associations. It is uncertain how well the changes in organizational and financial arrangements will meet the requirements of this client group in the long term.

5.2.3 WHAT TYPE OF PATIENT SHOULD LIVE IN WHAT TYPE OF ACCOMMODATION AND WHAT MAKES FOR A SUCCESSFUL PLACEMENT?

Despite the fact that clinical decisions about placement are made constantly in every rehabilitation and long-term care service, very little research has been carried out looking at the relationship between client characteristics, accommodation characteristics and the likelihood of successful placements. What research there is largely consists of descriptive reports on hostels and group homes (e.g. Ryan and Hewitt, 1976; Ryan and Wing, 1979; Pritlove, 1983; Jones, Robinson and Golightly, 1986), evaluation of individual projects (e.g. Wykes, 1983; Garety and Morris, 1984; Goldberg *et al.*, 1985; Gibbons and Butler, 1987), and evaluation of social environments (e.g. Ryan and Wing, 1979; Apte, 1968; Ryan and Hewitt, 1976; King, Raynes and Tizard, 1971; Garety and Morris, 1984; Segal and Moyles, 1979; Allen, Gillespie and Hall, 1989). These studies are interesting in their own right, and add to our knowledge, but there is still a very long way to go before we can plan with confidence the optimal living arrangements for people with severe and persistent psychiatric problems (Pritlove, 1983).

Given the important contribution which the quality of accommodation makes to overall quality of life for this client group (Waismann, 1988; Thapa and Rowland, 1989), this is rather a sorry state of affairs. Nevertheless, there are a few studies which can offer some valuable insights for the clinician trying to make decisions about an individual's accommodation, and these will be looked at below.

In clinical practice two aspects of a patient's behaviour are normally considered when decisions about accommodation are being made: level of functioning in daily living skills and degree of antisocial behaviour. It is these two factors which are measured on the REHAB scale (Hall and Baker, 1983) developed to guide decisions about the placement of patients who had been living on long-stay wards in psychiatric asylums. Although the authors of this scale report that level of functioning alone can be used to make decisions about placement (Baker and Hall, 1983), which probably reflects what happens in clinical practice (e.g. Carson, Croucher and Abrahamson, 1989), with the lowest functioning people being allocated to the most structured and supported accommodation, evidence is now emerging that degree of antisocial behaviour is the more important determinant of placement success (Zipple and Elkind, 1984; Clifford *et al.*, 1991; Conning & Brownlow, 1992). For example, Hill (1988) examined the relationship between factors about residents and hostels and the success of placements in a range of voluntary sector hostels for the long-term mentally ill. She found that, although hostels with more client-oriented attitudes rather than management-oriented attitudes took clients with disruptive behaviour, when things did not work out because of disruptive behaviour they ejected the client, and there was a lot of conflict about the departure between the hostel staff and the resident.

Even in hostel-wards set up to take the most disabled patients, disruptive behaviour is often not tolerated. For example, in Douglas House in Manchester, having a prior history of behavioural disturbance predicted difficulty in the behaviour being managed in the hostel-ward and consequent ejection (Creighton, Hyde and Farragher, 1991). Similarly, Gibbons (1986) found that the patients rejected from the hospital-hostel in Southampton were those who were 'aggressive, and prone to express and act on odd ideas. They posed more control problems and were felt to be too disturbed for other residents and too much of a risk in a hostel situated off the hospital campus and in the centre of the city'. The Maudsley hospital-hostel, in London, has proved to be much better at managing this group of patients (Wykes, 1983) perhaps because it is situated on the hospital site. Knowing that people with anti-social and disruptive behaviour are hard to place begs the question 'how can they be accommodated?'. This issue will be addressed in Chapter 6.

One way of getting round the problem of the accommodation of people with anti-social and disruptive behaviour may be to change the way that hostel staff respond to this behaviour. Moore, Kuipers and Ball (1992), suggest that high- and low-expressed emotion (EE) attitudes exist in professional carers, and that these attitudes affect the staff's behaviour towards patients. Staff with low-EE attitudes, despite dealing with difficult behaviour on a regular basis, were able to contain their own feelings when confronted by patients. They accepted the patients, empathized with the difficulties they were facing and valued their participation in working towards a programme of management. These are the very aspects of staff behaviour which generate workable treatment programmes (Isaacs and Bebbington, 1991) and which are likely to foster optimism in staff and independence in patients (Moore, Kuipers and Ball, 1992). Moore, Kuipers and Ball found that staff were most able to tolerate difficult behaviour when they believed it to be due to the patient's illness, rather than to difficulties in the patient's personality, and suggest that training should be geared towards helping staff to identify symptoms within an 'illness' model, particularly as helping relatives to do this has been an important part of their education (Berkowitz et al., 1984; Leff et al., 1982).

The degree of disruptive behaviour is unlikely to be the only determinant of successful placement in accommodation. Wykes and Dunn (1992) studied what happened to chronic patients over a 6-year period during which time there was a partial hospital closure. Although 71% were able to move to more independent residential settings, including 38% who moved to live in their own accommodation often with little support from the psychiatric services, those who were unable to do so had performed poorly on a response processing measure. They argue that their response processing task taps a cognitive dysfunction which is central to schizophrenia, and that degree of cognitive dysfunction is a significant predictor of the level of care needed by the client.

One might also expect that resident satisfaction with a placement would be related to its success. Residents appear to prefer client-oriented accommodation (Segal and Moyles, 1979; Hill, 1988) although staff in management-oriented accommodation are perceived as more helpful (Hill, 1988).

5.2.4 SHOULD PATIENTS WHO ARE MOVING FROM ONE TYPE OF ACCOMMODATION TO ANOTHER BE PREPARED FOR THE MOVE AND, IF SO, HOW?

Again, there is little or no research into how to prepare patients for accommodation moves or if this should be done, although common sense and common humanity suggest that it must be advantageous. When somebody is moving, particularly if the move is from a psychiatric ward to a house, several questions spring to mind.

- Who is the person moving with – do they know the residents and staff?
- What will the person be expected to do when they move – are there skills which should be acquired?
- What changes will be effected in the individual's life by the move?

In the Southampton rehabilitation and long-term care service, a National Demonstration Service, the staff preparing to move long-stay residents from the hospital site to a hospital-hostel in the centre of Southampton have developed an extensive package of preparation for the residents, who were chosen with the aid of the Community Placement Questionnaire (Clifford et al., 1991). Although there is no research evidence that the preparation package has helped the staff and residents effect a successful move, or which particular elements of it have been important, the staff are committed to it and it covers all the questions raised above. The residents were selected from three or four wards and moved initially to an empty house on the hospital site. This provided the opportunity for staff and residents to get to know one another and to get used to living and working in a hospital-hostel before having to cope with the move off the hospital site. While still on the hospital site a number of activities were carried out to prepare everyone for the move. Firstly, and importantly, residents were kept informed of the progress of the move. They were taken to see their new home, so that they would see the progress in the building works as it took place. A video was made for those who refused to go and look. The environment around the new hostel was also explored, for example, finding out the locations of local cafes, banks and clubs. As part of the process of keeping people informed, there was a handbook of useful information written by staff and residents, which included information on buses, fares, the post office and so on. Opportunities were provided for residents to learn and practise skills which would be appropriate in the new setting: budgeting, road safety, self-medication, use of cafes, using banks and building societies, using cash machines. Residents were educated about racial issues and sexuality. Groups were run about looking back and moving forward, encouraging the residents to explore their recollections about the past and their thoughts about moving; and how to say goodbye. The staff had to introduce the various activities gradually because many of the residents became upset at the thought of being expected to do so much. But the aim of the preparation package was to make residents familiar with as much as possible about their new homes and their new routines before having to cope with the move off the 'safe' hospital site.

The Netherne Rehabilitation Service in East Surrey has compiled a checklist which helps ensure that all the necessary tasks are completed just prior to a patient moving out of hospital.

1. Liaison
- Involvement/consultation with the rehabilitee
- Communication with the family/carer
- Informing relevant people of the moving date
- Contact with key personnel
- Social Report for the Housing Association if necessary

2. Accommodation
- Viewing the accommodation with the rehabilitee
- Checking safe use by the rehabilitee of the cooker, heaters, meters, door locks etc.
- Checking that the water, gas, electricity, heating are in order and so on for the moving day
- Checking that the furniture/furnishings are in order
- Acquisition and transport of additional items

3. Money
- Have relevant benefits been applied for?
- Are medical certificates/rent/benefit documentation ready?
- Rent, how much/how to be paid
- Money and food for immediate needs
- Visit to DSS on the moving day

4. Work
- Daytime occupation/work
- Referrals if necessary

5. Transport
- For the rehabilitee plus belongings on the moving day
- For belongings from the previous accommodation, if any

6. Locality
- Registration with GP/dentist etc.
- Familiarization with the local area – GP surgery, bus stops, shops, launderette, phone booths etc.
- Practice in use of buses, shops, money etc. if needed
- Provision of local maps, bus/train timetables

7. Follow-up
- Medication to take away; who prescribes/provides in future?
- Personal discharge card (giving contact numbers and names)
- Outpatient appointments
- Referrals

8. Other
- Clothing
- What to do in an emergency

Many people with long-term and severe mental health problems find it very difficult to cope with change. They may become anxious at the thought of impending change, and/or after the change has taken place, resulting in an increase in their psychiatric symptomatology. Of course, anxiety about change, and difficulty coping with change or new situations, are normal human experiences. One way that people deal with this in every day life is to find out as much as possible about the new and unfamiliar situation before it is experienced, so that it becomes more familiar, and one can learn how to deal with those aspects of it which might be difficult. It seems reasonable to assume that such an approach will be useful to people with long-term psychiatric problems too.

5.3 LEISURE AND SOCIALIZING

The term 'leisure' usually means engaging in spare time pleasurable activities which may be shared with others, in contrast with 'idleness', which denotes doing nothing, often in isolation. Training in the use of time for recreation and socializing is an important rehabilitation intervention which, when successful, contributes to social adjustment, enjoyment and personal fulfilment. Moreover, there is a good deal of evidence that inactivity and social isolation contribute to increased disability.

Years of illness and hospitalization often leave disabled people ill-equipped for this area of community living, which others take for granted; a disabled person may also lack the necessary motivation, knowledge, skill and money to take up hobbies and interests and to develop social networks. Self-report time budget schedules for weekdays and Sundays were used as part of a rehabilitation service's follow-up study (Collis and Ekdawi, 1984); waking time divided into obligatory activities, comprising work and subsistence (household and personal care) activities and discretionary (leisure) ones. Discretionary activities generally depend on a number of variables including age, place, family roles, income and social class, as well as on subjective factors such as preference, taste and knowledge.

In the study, discretionary activities tended to be of three types: hobbies and interests, socializing and doing nothing. Although the first two were not mutually exclusive, in practice few rehabilitees shared their leisure interests with others. Doing nothing consisted of resting, day-time sleeping, just sitting, waiting (usually for the next meal) and passively listening to the radio as a background noise.

Rehabilitees resident in hospital generally spent more time doing nothing than did those living in community settings. Overall, both the hospital and the community rehabilitation programmes helped the individuals to make better use of their leisure time, although it was unclear whether this resulted in personally fulfilling activities rather than 'just filling the empty hours'. Interviews carried out with relatives of the same group showed that many were dissatisfied with the rehabilitees' use of leisure time as this frequently depended on the family stimulating them and, as a result, relatives' own social life, holidays and retirement plans were restricted. These findings echoed those in other studies, notably that by Stevens (1972) on the dependence of community patients on their elderly relatives.

In the case of people with severe levels of disability and whose long-term illnesses led to loss of contact with families and friends, this dependence is commonly transferred to statutory services. Although, ideally, disabled people should use as many community public facilities as possible, they often need special medical and social supports (Bennett and Morris, 1991). Of the day patients who regularly attended a hospital unit for many years, there was a 'fringe group' who made little or no intimate contact with other patients or with staff; however, in spite of their apparent social unengagement, they needed friendly, undemanding contact. A more socially engaged group experienced difficulties in getting close to anyone and, although some had confidants, they felt lonely (Mitchell and Birley, 1983). The unengaged group included more single men with a diagnosis of schizophrenia; their social characteristics were similar to those of the severely disabled long-stay patients described by Morgan (1979), some of whom never spoke to their companions, nor even knew their names.

This apparently very low level of socialization was also found in a cohort of 489 long-stay patients in another study, where three groups were identified. The social interactions of the first group were passive and limited to simple greetings or non-verbal interchanges. Their communication skills were poor, with a restricted range of emotional expression, and they often relied on exchange of goods and services to create 'as intimate a bond as the sharing of confidences'. In the second group, there was an 80% chance of regular conversations occurring, while in the third only non-verbal transactions were found (Leff et al., 1990). These examples clearly show the wide spectrum of deficits in socializing skills which inevitably affect the use of discretionary time, and they point to the enormous range of provisions needed.

There are many factors, often co-existing, which cause and perpetuate the problems experienced by disabled people in the use of their discretionary time.

- Difficulties in pursuing leisure activities and in socializing may be present premorbidly, sometimes as a personality characteristic.
- Negative symptoms of schizophrenia, which include social withdrawal, slowness, poverty of speech, lack of spontaneity and blunting or inappropriateness of emotional expression and responsiveness, severely limit social interaction.
- Anxiety and indecisiveness, often associated with disability (Seeman, Littman and Plummer, 1982) create difficulties in engaging with others and in attempting unstructured, and therefore unpredictable and anxiety-provoking, activities.
- Antipsychotic medication may produce extrapyramidal side-effects, including reduction in non-verbal expressivity which, in turn, elicits negative responses from others.
- One of the hallmarks of some institutional environments, where social stimulation is minimal, is their tendency to enforce and reinforce inactivity and idleness.
- Long-term illness and hospitalization vastly diminish the chance of reviving old contacts and friendships; a well-motivated man, for example, who tried to rejoin his amateur dramatics club found that he 'felt like a total stranger'. Such efforts at re-integration in a social group are further undermined by feelings of stigma.
- The risks of high levels of social stimulation inherent in some socializing and recreational activities could arouse unpleasant feelings or even precipitate symptom relapse; in this context, social withdrawal may be a protective strategy.
- Insufficient financial resources may already restrict spending on essential subsistence needs and could make it impossible, for example, to join or travel to a club, or to develop a hobby.

Rehabilitation training in the constructive use of leisure time is usually based on a combination of three approaches.

1. **Behavioural skills training** in this area is important, but may present difficulties because, by definition, discretionary activities tend to be unstructured. Social functioning, in general, comprises a number of semi-independent systems (Strauss and Carpenter, 1977); a person who functions well in his role as a worker, for example, may flounder in less structured social gatherings. It is useful to bear in mind that while role performance requires a variety of skills, competence in specific skills by itself does not guarantee adequate performance (Appelo et al., 1992). For instance, the discrete skills of travelling, buying an admission ticket and being able to swim do not necessarily add up to global competence in undertaking the role of a leisure centre user. Successful behavioural training often includes counselling (Wallace et al., 1992).

2. **Counselling** is fruitful in the sphere of leisure education. It includes an exploration of the individual's satisfaction and dissatisfactions with his life-style and his willingness to change, as well as his interests and preferences. Techniques to overcome constraints are considered and an action plan is designed and agreed (Searle, 1971).

3. **Assistance in developing social networks** which are consistent with the person's interests and where opportunities to form supportive contacts and friendships are offered may well prove rewarding (Thornicroft and Breackey, 1991). It is easier to embark on and to maintain a leisure activity if it is shared with one or more partners; being involved with a reference group, for example in a day unit, may be a bridge towards forming wider networks. This is, however, a slow step by step process which requires much support; its successful management depends on 'walking a tight rope' between over- and under-stimulation (Shepherd, 1988).

In conclusion, there is sufficient evidence to show that the use of discretionary time has a powerful influence on social adjustment and the quality of life; in spite of its complexity, such training should be considered as an essential component of rehabilitation programmes.

REFERENCES

Abdul-Hamid, W. and McCarthy, M. (1989) Community psychiatric care for homeless people in inner London. *Health Trends*, **21**, 67–69.

Acharya, S., Ekdawi, M.Y., Gallagher, L. and Glaister, B. (1982) Day hospital rehabilitation: a six year study. *Social Psychiatry*, **17**, 1–5.

Allen, C.I., Gillespie, R. and Hall, J.N. (1989) A comparison of practices, attitudes and interactions in two established units for people with a psychiatric disability. *Psychological Medicine*, **19**, 459–467.

Anthony, W.A., Cohen, M.R. and Danley, K.S. (1988) The psychiatric rehabilitation approach as applied to vocational rehabilitation, in *Vocational Rehabilitation of Persons with Prolonged Mental Illness*, (ed. W.A. Anthony), Baltimore, Johns Hopkins University Press.

Appelo, M.T., Woonings, F.M.J., Van Nieuwenhuisen, C.J. *et al.* (1992) Specific skills and social competence in schizophrenia. *Acta Psychiatrica Scandinavica*, **85**, 419–422.

Apte, R.Z. (1968) *Halfway houses: a new dilemma in institutional care. Occasional Papers in Social Administration*, No. 27, G. Bells & Sons, London.

Baker, R.D. and Hall, J.N. (1983) *REHAB: User's Manual*, Vine Publishing, Aberdeen.

Bates, P. and Walsh, M. (1989) *Empty Premises – Empty Promises*, Nottingham. Benefits Research Unit, Occasional Papers, 1/89.

Bennett, D. and Morris, I. (1991) Support and rehabilitation, in *Theory and Practice of Psychiatric Rehabilitation*, (eds F.N. Watts and D.H. Bennett), John Wiley & Sons, Chichester.

Berkowitz, R., Eberlein-Fries, R., Kuipers, L. and Leff, J. (1984) Educating relatives about schizophrenia. *Schizophrenia Bulletin*, **10**, 418–429.

Brenner, M.H. (1979) Mortality and the national economy: a review, and the experience of England and Wales. *Lancet*, **ii**, 568–573.

Brenner, M.A. (1987) Relation of economic and social well-being, 1950–1980. *Social Science Medicine*, **25**, 183–196.

Carson, J., Croucher, P. and Abrahamson, D. (1989) *Using REHAB in Rehabilitation and Resettlement*. Paper presented at a symposium sponsored by the British Psychological Society, Dec. 20.

Chatel, J. and Joe, B. (1975) Psychiatry in Spain – past and present. *American Journal of Psychiatry*, **132**, 1182–1186.

Clifford, P., Charman, A., Webb, Y. *et al.* (1991) Planning for community care: the community placement questionnaire. *British Journal of Clinical Psychology*, **30**, 193–221.

Collis, M. and Ekdawi, M.Y. (1984) Social adjustment in rehabilitation. *International Journal of Rehabilitation Research*, **7**, 259–272.

Conning, A.M. and Brownlow, J. (1992) Determining suitability of placement for long-stay psychiatric inpatients. *Hospital and Community Psychiatry*, **43**(7), 709–712.

Conning, A.M. and Rowland, L.A. (1991) Where do people with longterm mental health problems live? A comparison of the sexes. *British Journal of Psychiatry*, **158** (suppl. 10), 80–84.

Creighton, F.J., Hyde, C.E. and Farragher, B. (1991) Douglas House: Seven Years' Experience of a Community hostel ward. *British Journal of Psychiatry*, **159**, 500–504.

Daniel, W.W. (1974) *A National Survey of the Unemployed*, Political and Economic Planning, London.

Daniels, D.N. (1966) New concepts of rehabilitation as applied to hiring the mentally restored. *Community Mental Health Journal*, **2**, 197–201.

Department of Health (1990) *National Health Service and Community Care Act*, HMSO, London.

Dickey, B., Cannon, N.L., McGuire, T. and Gudeman, J.G. (1986) The quarterway house: a two-year cost study of an experimental residential programme. *Hospital and Community Psychiatry*, **37**(11), 1136–1143.

Early, D.F. (1960) The Industrial Therapy Organisation (Bristol). *Lancet*, **ii**, 754–757.

Ekdawi, M.Y. (1966) Changes in the ward behaviour of severely disabled schizophrenic patients: a four years study. *British Journal of Psychiatry*, **112**, 265–267.

Ekdawi, M.Y. (1972) The Netherne Resettlement Unit results of ten years. *British Journal of Psychiatry*, **121**, 417–424.

Ekdawi, M.Y. (1981) Counselling in rehabilitation, in *Handbook of Psychiatric Rehabilitation Practice*, (eds. J.K. Wing and B. Morris), Oxford University Press, London.

Ekdawi, M.Y. (1989) Work at Netherne – a service responding to change. *Psychiatric Bulletin*, **13**, 30–32.

Falloon, I.R. and Marshall, G.N. (1983) Residential care and social behaviour: a study of rehabilitation needs. *Psychological Medicine*, **13**, 341–347.

Floyd, M., Gregory, E., Murray, H. and Welchman, R. (1983) *Schizophrenia* and Employment. Tavistock Institute of Human Relations Occasional Paper No. 5, Tavistock Publications, London.

Freudenberg, R.K. (1960) *Work Therapy in Psychiatric Hospitals*. Maudsley Bequest Lecture, February 1966.

Garety, P. (1988) Housing, in *Community Care in Practice*, (eds A. Lavender and F. Holloway), John Wiley & Sons, Chichester, Ch. 8.

Garety, P.A. and Morris, I. (1984) A new unit for long-stay psychiatric patients: organisation, attitudes and quality of care. *Psychological Medicine*, **14**, 183–192.

Gibbons, J. (1986) Care of 'new' long-stay patients in a District General Hospital Psychiatric Unit: the first two years of a hospital-hostel. *Acta Psychiatrica Scandinavica*, **73**, 582–588.

Gibbons, J.S. and Butler, J.P. (1987) Quality of life for 'new' long-stay psychiatric in-patients: the effects of moving to a hostel. *British Journal of Psychiatry*, **151**, 347–354.

Gloag, D. (1985) Occupational rehabilitation and return to work: 2. Psychiatric disability. *British Medical Journal*, **290**, 1201.

Goldberg, D.P., Bridges, K., Cooper, W. *et al.* (1985) Douglas House, a new type of hostel ward for chronic psychotic patients. *British Journal of Psychiatry*, **147**, 383–388.

Griffiths, R (1988) *Community Care: Agenda for Action*, HMSO, London.

Grove, B. (1989) Integration into the working world. *Psychiatric Bulletin*, **13**, 28–30.

Hall, J.N. and Baker, R.D. (1983) *REHAB*, Vine Publishing, Aberdeen.

Hartley, J. (1980) Psychological approaches to unemployment. *Bulletin of the British Psychological Society*, **32**, 309–314.

Higgs, R. (1981) Unemployment in my practice: Walworth. *British Medical Journal*, **283**, 532.

Hill, B.A. (1988) Factors influencing satisfaction and successful placement in hostels for people with a long-term psychiatric disability. University of London, MSc Thesis.

House of Commons Social Services Committee (1985) *Community Care with Special Reference to Adult Mentally Ill and Mentally Handicapped People*. Second Report from the Social Services Committee, HMSO, London.

Isaacs, A.D. and Bebbington, P.E. (1991) Strategies for the management of severe psychiatric illness in the community. *International Review of Psychiatry*, **3**, 71–82.

Jahoda, M., Lazenfeld, P.F. and Zeisel, H. (1972) *Marienthal, the Sociology of an Unemployed Community*, Tavistock Publications, London.

Jones, K., Robinson, M. and Golightly, M. (1986) Long-term psychiatric patients in the community. *British Journal of Psychiatry*, **149**, 537–540.

Jones, M. (1956) Industrial rehabilitation of mental patients still in hospital. *Lancet*, **3**, 985–986.

Kay, A. and Legg, C. (1986) *Discharged to the Community: a Review of Housing and Support in London for People Leaving Psychiatric Care*, Good Practices in Mental Health, London.

King, R.D., Raynes, N.V. and Tizard, J. (1971) *Patterns of Residential Care*, Routledge and Kegan Paul, London.

Lamb, H.R. (1982) *Treating the Long-term Mentally Ill*, Jossey-Bass, San Francisco.

Lang, E. and Rio, J. (1989) A psychiatric rehabilitation vocational program in a private psychiatric hospital: the New York Hospital-Cornell Medical Center, in *Psychiatric Rehabilitation Programs – Putting Theory into Practice,* (eds M.D. Farkas and W.A. Anthony), Johns Hopkins University Press, Baltimore.

Leff, J., Kuipers, L., Berkowitz, R., Eberlein-Fries, R. and Sturgeon, D. (1982) A controlled trial of social intervention in the families of schizophrenic patients. *British Journal of Psychiatry,* **141,** 121–134.

Leff, J., O'Driscoll, C., Dayson, D. *et al.* (1990) The TAPS Project: 5. The structure of social-network data obtained from long-stay patients. *British Journal of Psychiatry,* **157,** 848–852.

Lehman, A.F., Ward., N.C. and Linn, L.S. (1982) Chronic mental patients: the quality of life issue. *American Journal of Psychiatry,* **139,** 1271–1276.

Lodge Patch, L.C. (1971) Homeless men in London: I. Demographic findings in the lodgings house sample. *British Journal of Psychiatry,* **118,** 313–317.

Marshall, M. (1989) Collected and neglected: are Oxford hostels for the homeless filling up with disabled psychiatric patients? *British Medical Journal,* **299,** 706–709.

Miles, A. (1971) Long-stay schizophrenic patients in hospital workshops. *British Journal of Psychiatry,* **119,** 611–620.

Mills, N. (1991) The structure of work environments in psychiatric rehabilitation. *Psychiatric Bulletin,* **15,** 69–72.

Mitchell, S.F. and Birley, J.L.T. (1983) The use of ward support by psychiatric patients in the community. *British Journal of Psychiatry,* **142,** 9–15.

Moore, E., Kuipers, L. and Ball, R. (1992) Staff-patient relationships in the care of the long-term adult mentally ill. *Social Psychiatry and Psychiatric Epidemiology,* **27,** 28–34.

Morgan, R. (1979) Conversations with chronic schizophrenic patients. *British Journal of Psychiatry,* **134,** 187–194.

Morgan, R. (1983) Indusrial therapy in the mental hospital, in *Theory and Practice of Psychiatric Rehabilitation,* (eds F.N. Watts and D.H. Bennett), John Wiley & Sons, Chichester.

Morgan, R. and Cheadle, J. (1981) *Psychiatric Rehabilitation.* Surbiton, National Schizophrenia Fellowship.

Moser, K., Goldblatt, P.O., Fox, A.J. and Jones, D.R. (1987) Unemployment and mortality: comparison of the 1971 and 1981 longitudinal study census samples. *British Medical Journal,* **294,** 86–90.

Mowbray, C.T., Greenfield, A. and Fereddolino, P.P. (1992) An analysis of treatment services provided in group homes for adults labelled mentally ill. *Journal of Nervous and Mental Disease,* **180**(9), 551–559.

Nordentoft, M., Knudsen, H.C. and Schulsinger, F. (1992) Housing conditions and residential needs of psychiatric patients in Copenhagen. *Acta Psychiatrica Scandinavica,* **85,** 385–389.

Patrick, M., Higgit, A. and Holloway, F. (1989) Changes in an inner city psychiatric inpatient service following bed losses: a follow-up of the East Lambeth 1986 Survey. *Health Trends,* **21,** 121–123.

Platt, S. and Kretman, N. (1984) Trends in parasuicide and unemployment among men in Edinburgh 1968–82. *British Medical Journal,* **289,** 1029–1032.

Priest, R.G. (1970), Homeless men, a USA–UK comparison. *Proceedings of the Royal Society of Medicine,* **63,** 441–445.

Priest, R.G. (1971) The Edinburgh homeless, a psychiatric survey. *American Journal of Psychotherapy*, **25**, 194–213.

Pritlove, J. (1983) Accommodation without resident staff for ex-psychiatric patients. *British Journal of Social Work*, **13**, 75–92.

Rapoport, R.N. (1960) *Community as Doctor: New Perspectives on a Therapeutic Community*, Tavistock Publications, London.

Rowland, L.A. (1990) *De-institutionalization, Politics and its Consequences in the United Kingdom*. Paper presented at El Rehabilitación del Paciente Mental Crónico en la Comunidad, Junta de Andalucia/Universidad Internacional Mendez Pelayo, Seville.

Rowland, L.A. and Perkins, R.E. (1988) *Health Trends*, **20**, 75–79.

Rowland, L.A., Zeelan, J. and Waismann, L.C. (1992) Patterns of service for the long-term mentally ill in Europe. *British Journal of Clinical Psychology*, **31**, 405–417.

Ryan, P. and Hewitt, S.H. (1976) A pilot study of hostels for the mentally ill. *Social Work Today*, **6**, 774–778.

Ryan, P. and Wing, J.K. (1979) Patterns of residential care: a study of hostels and group homes used by 4 local authorities to support the mentally ill in the community, in *Alternative Patterns of Residential Care for the Discharged Psychiatric Patient*, (ed. R. Olsen), BASW, Birmingham.

Schwartz, D.B. (1976) Expanding a sheltered workshop to replace nonpaying patient jobs. *Hospital and Community Psychiatry*, **27**, 98–101.

Scott, B. (1982) *Mental Illness and Employability*. Washington, DC, President's Committee on Employment of the Handicapped.

Searle, M.S (1971) Leisure education in a day hospital: the effects on selected social-psychological variables. *Canadian Journal of Community Mental Health*, **1012**, 95–109.

Seeman, M.V., Littman, S.K. and Plummer, E. (1982) *Living and Working with Schizophrenia*, Open University Press, Milton Keynes.

Segal, S.P. and Moyles, F.W. (1979) Management style and institutional dependency in sheltered care. *Social Psychiatry*, **14**, 159–165.

Shepherd, G. (1984) *Institutional Care and Rehabilitation*. Longmans, Harlow.

Shepherd, G. (1988) Practical aspects of the management of negative symptoms. *International Journal of Mental Health*, **16**, 75–97.

Smith, R. (1987) *Unemployment and Health*, Oxford University Press, Oxford.

Stevens, B. (1972) Dependence of schizophrenic patients on elderly relatives. *Psychological Medicine*, **2**, 17–23.

Strauss, J.S. and Carpenter, W.T. (1977) Prediction of outcome and its predictors. *Archives of General Psychiatry*, **34**, 159–167.

Thapa, K. and Rowland, L.A. (1989) Quality of life perspectives in long-term care: Staff and patient perceptions. *Acta Psychiatrica Scandinavica*, **80**, 267–271.

Thornicroft, G. and Breackey, W.R. (1991) Improving social networks of the long-term mentally ill. *British Journal of Psychiatry*, **159**, 245–249.

Waismann, L.C. (1988) Needs and other motivational processes in long-term psychiatric patients in an era of community care. University of London. PhD Thesis.

Wallace, C.J., Liberman, R.P., MacKain, S.J. *et al.* (1992) Effectiveness and replicability of modules for teaching social and instrumental skills to the severely mentally ill. *American Journal of Psychiatry*, **149**, 654–658.

Wansbrough, N. and Cooper, P. (1980) *Open Employment After Mental Illness*. Tavistock Publications, London.

Warr, P. (1985) Twelve questions about unemployment and health, in *New Approaches to Economic Life*, (eds. R. Roberts, R. Finnegan and D. Gallie), Manchester University Press, Manchester.

Warr, P. (1987) *Work, Unemployment and Mental Health*, Oxford University Press, Oxford.

Watts, F.N. (1978) A Study of work behaviour in a psychiatric rehabilitation unit. *British Journal of Social and Clinical Psychology*, **17**, 85–92.

Watts, F.N. (1983) Employment, in *Theory and Practice of Psychiatric Rehabilitation* (eds. F.N. Watts and D.H. Bennett), John Wiley & Sons, Chichester.

Weinman, B. and Kleiner, R.J. (1978) The impact of community living and community member intervention on the adjustment of the chronic psychiatric patient, in *Alternatives to Mental Hospital Treatment*, (eds L.I. Stein and M.A. Test), Plenum Press, New York.

Wing, J.K. (1966) Social and psychological changes in a rehabilitation unit. *Social Psychiatry*, **1**, 21–28.

Wing, J.K., Bennett, D.H. and Denham, J. (1964) *Industrial Rehabilitation of Long-stay Schizophrenic Patients*. Medical Research Council Memo No. 42. HMSO, London.

Wing, J.K. and Brown, G.W. (1970) *Institutionalism and Schizophrenia*, Cambridge University Press, Cambridge.

Wing, J.K. and Freudenberg, R.K. (1961) The response of severely ill chronic schizophrenic patients to social stimulation. *American Journal of Psychiatry*, **118**, 311–322.

Wing, J.K. and Furlong, R. (1986) A Haven for the severely disabled within the context of a comprehensive psychiatric community service. *British Journal of Psychiatry*, **149**, 449–457.

Wykes, T. (1983) A follow-up of 'new' long-stay patients in Camberwell, 1977–82. *Psychological Medicine*, **13**, 659–662.

Wykes, T. and Dunn, G. (1992) Cognitive deficit and prediction of rehabilitation success in a chronic psychiatric group. *Psychological Medicine*, **22**, 389–398.

Zipple, A.M. and Elkind, M. (1984) The role of client level of functioning in residential placement decisions. *Psychosocial Rehabilitation Journal*, **7**, 56–65.

Resettlement

6

In Chapter 2, we saw that an early definition of rehabilitation encompassed the concept of resettlement, using employment off the hospital site as a stepping stone towards leaving the hospital altogether. Although resettlement aimed 'to restore the patient to the most satisfactory life of which he is capable, despite his disabilities' (Bennett, Folkard and Nicholson, 1961), hopes were high that the majority of people living in psychiatric asylums would improve to the point at which they might be able to live and work in 'normal' settings. Although the concept of resettlement is no longer fashionable, the deinstitutionalization movement has raised two dilemmas:

- are there some people who cannot survive without the type of sheltered environment which was provided in the psychiatric asylums?
- what should be the future role of hospitals in the care of people with long-term and severe mental health problems?

There is now considerable agreement that, despite effective rehabilitation and long-term care programmes, there remain substantial numbers of people 'with residual disabilities severe enough to require, in the long-term, psychiatric services equivalent to those currently offered in hospitals' (O'Driscoll, Marshall and Reed, 1990). The evidence for this has come from several sources. Firstly, despite the development of services to replace the psychiatric asylums, this has not led to a reduction in the number of long-stay admissions to hospital beds in many services (for example, Fryers and Wooff, 1989; O'Driscoll, Marshall and Reed, 1990; Clifford *et al.* 1991b; Lawrence, Copas and Cooper, 1991).

There is little evidence that the very considerable extensions of 'community' services in the last two decades have materially affected the use of in-patient care: they have not reduced admission, not changed the distribution of length of stay, and not reduced the numbers of people admitted for at least a year (Fryers and Wooff, 1989).

Secondly, some patients have not survived in provisions which have been set up to replace the psychiatric asylums and so have returned permanently to hospital. For example, Thornicroft and Gooch (1991) found that 6% of their group of 347 hospital leavers were readmitted permanently to hospital. Even though many districts have set up hostel-wards or hospital-hostels to cater for the most disabled long-term clients, some of their residents have had to return to hospital (for example, Gibbons, 1986; Garety, Afele and Isaacs, 1988; Creighton, Hyde and Farragher, 1991). Thirdly, it is a common experience that the patients left in psychiatric asylums once a closure programme has begun are those who are the most difficult to place (Carson and Shaw, 1989; Clifford et al., 1991b; Dayson and Gooch, 1991), suggesting difficulty in knowing how to plan for these patients who need innovative services (Dayson and Gooch, 1991).

What types of problems are these 'difficult to place' patients likely to have? There seems to be general agreement that they have severe behavioural problems (Gudeman and Shore, 1984; Gibbons, 1986; Wing and Furlong, 1986; Clifford et al., 1991a; Creighton, Hyde and Farragher, 1991) which raise issues both about their management and their public acceptability. Some (e.g. Wing and Furlong, 1986; Clifford et al., 1991b) argue that there is also a separate group of patients who are amongst the last to leave long-stay wards who may or may not have behavioural problems but whose main problems are their poor living skills and high levels of physical disability; and Wykes and Dunn (1992) have found that poor response processing predicts difficulty in survival without hospital-type care.

This leaves the question of how people are to be cared for once the psychiatric asylums have closed. The concept of hostel-wards and hospital-hostels was developed in order to cater for these clients but as has already been discussed, there has been mixed success. The original idea of the hostel-ward, as developed at 111 Denmark Hill, at the Maudsley Hospital, London, was that the house should be placed on the edge of the hospital site so that the resources of the hospital could be called upon if and when necessary (Wykes, 1982). Attempts to emulate this facility have created the hospital-hostel, which has a similar structure of care to the hostel-ward, but the building is usually placed in a domestic street away from the hospital site (Goldberg et al., 1985; Gibbons, 1986). Evidence is beginning to accumulate that whereas hospital-hostels placed away from the hospital site sometimes have difficulty in accommodating people with severe behavioural disturbance (Gibbons, 1986; Creighton, Hyde and Farragher, 1991) such residents can be managed when the hostel is on the hospital site and short admissions to a more secure environment are possible in times of crisis (Garety, Afele and Isaacs, 1988; Kingdon *et al.*, 1991). Garety, Afele and Isaacs (1988) claim that 111 Denmark Hill has only rejected people who have multiple physical disabilities, as well as multiple mental disabilities, and that their failures have occurred when residents have discharged themselves from the hostel in an unplanned way, leading to failure to survive in the accommodation to which they have then moved.

Although this suggests that it is proximity to the hospital site which makes the management and tolerance of severe behavioural disturbance possible, at this stage the evidence is not conclusive. Neither is it known what it might be about this proximity which is important. For example, is it that the residents can get out of the hostel to attend daytime activities on the hospital site? Or that even if they do not take part in activities, the day facilities on the hospital site provide a place to go, where friends can be met? Or are the grounds of the hospital themselves important, providing a protective barrier from the outside world, inside which unusual behaviour is tolerated? Or is it that staff are able to tolerate more difficult behaviour because help from the rest of the hospital is so near at hand? Or perhaps there is something unique about the regime in 111 Denmark Hill which has not quite been captured in other places. Unfortunately, the evidence does not allow one to do more than speculate.

Wing and Furlong (1986) have suggested an adaptation to the hostel-ward model to cater for a range of patients who are difficult to place, as well as the groups discussed above. Their Haven Community concept consists of four core hostels placed on the edge of the hospital site: one for younger persistently disturbed people plus some respite beds for short admissions; one for long-term severely disabled people with physical problems also such as epilepsy or Huntington's chorea; one for those who tend, if unsupervized, to wander without regard to danger; and the fourth for frail elderly people with long-standing functional psychiatric disorders. In addition they argue that there should be a range of houses and flatlets with a lower degree of supervision 'so that maximum independence can be developed and maintained in those whose disorders necessitate lengthy care, e.g. those with unpredictable behaviour, those detained because of legal offences and those with major dependency problems.

This accommodation constitutes the Haven, but

in addition, linked to the Haven but scattered among the local housing estate would be peripheral group homes and supervised apartments, set up in association with the local authority or charitable organizations, in order to provide for 'graduates' who still need various degrees of Haven support and also for people who are a rung or two up the ladder but highly vulnerable to relapse (Wing and Furlong, 1986).

This arrangement should allow ease of movement into and out of the Community and facilitate continuity of care by maintaining contact with those who move out of the Community. They also envisage opportunities for recreation, daytime occupation and work both on and off the Community site. Wing and Furlong argue that one of the major advantages of maintaining a 'core' on the hospital site is that it provides space where people can wander in private and where those with odd gestures, demeanour or behaviour will not be ridiculed or arrested.

Whether or not maintaining some services for the most disabled and disturbed patients on the hospital site will be a necessity, or an advantage, remains to be seen. In many Districts the only possible hospital site will be the District General Hospital which may have other disadvantages (Gibbons, 1986) and which is unlikely to provide the space to wander in private required by Wing and Furlong (1986). At the moment the continued admissions to long-stay beds (Fryers and Wooff, 1989; O'Driscoll, Marshall and Reed, 1990; Clifford et al., 1991b) suggest that in many cases the alternative services are not providing for the functions which these beds served.

Thornicroft and Bebbington (1989) have identified those functions of psychiatric hospitals which they believe to be impaired, eroded, or vulnerable in the alterantive service provision on offer. These include protection of patients from exploitation, respite for the family, haven/asylum for the patient, secure provision for involuntary patients, occupation and vocational rehabilitation, shelter, nutrition, basic income and clothing, job security for staff, segregation from society of deviant or dangerous members, economies of scale, segregation within psychiatry of less attractive patients and structured roles and identities for staff and patients. This is not to say that such functions cannot be reprovided, but one will have to think more creatively and pay attention to some of the less obvious functions of psychiatric hospitals if the new forms of care are to be successful.

The debate continues about whether, and in what form, hospital provision for long-term accommodation should continue. Long-term accommodation has been discussed in Chapter 5, but what about shorter admissions for domestic, social or psychiatric crises? Bachrach (1980) has argued that good services for people with long-term psychiatric disabilities are tied in some manner to a complement of hospital beds. Data from the District Services Centre (DSC), Bethlem Royal and Maudsley Special Health Authority, a 'community care' service which has been operating for over 10 years, will serve to illustrate the use to which such beds can be put. The DSC looks after approximately 350 long-term patients, and yet has only 34 hospital beds. Rowland, Perkins and Bennett (1987) found that during the first 5 years of the DSC being open, there was a steady decrease in the mean number of beds occupied per night from 30.9 in 1982 to 26.4 in 1986, suggesting that the service's ability to maintain people outside hospital had improved, or at least that the service was not gradually accumulating an increasing number of people who required long-term hospital care. However, Rowland, Perkins and Bennett (1987) also suggested that the service could not operate with less than 34 beds because at some points during each year all the beds were in use. The beds which were not occupied by long admissions provided the facility to admit people for brief periods, often as little as one night, which seemed to be a crucial part of maintaining some people 'in the community'.

Rowland, Perkins and Bennett (1987) conclude that the availability of beds for such brief admissions is an essential part of any service which is attempting to maintain long-term patients in the community. Their study also provides useful information about the range of uses to which beds attached to a long-term care service are likely to be put. They found that the beds served four quite distinct groups of patients: there were about nine 'new long-stay' patients waiting for a place in the hostel-ward; there were medium-term admissions of people who stayed for several months and who were preparing for accommodation outside hospital. There were many brief admissions of people who stayed from one night to several weeks, admitted in crisis or to prevent some crisis occurring; and there were one or two people at any one time who required 24-hour care in a closed setting because they were floridly disturbed and at risk of, for example, suicide.

Talbott and Glick (1986) have also outlined the reasons why hospitalization may sometimes be necessary for long-term patients, although they emphasize that hospitalization should usually be brief. The reasons they suggest include:

- re-evaluation of diagnosis and functioning, where the patient's functioning in the community may indicate he or she is not receiving the appropriate level of care;
- re-equilibration of medication where either too much medication has been given so the person is not performing the social coping functions necessary to community survival, or too little medication is indicated by, perhaps, the re-emergence of psychotic symptoms;

- to effect changes in treatment plans, such as moving from one community support element to another;
- when the patient cannot be managed outside hospital because he or she is overtly psychotic, homicidal or suicidal, or presents a danger to self or others;
- when the patient requires treatment that is not easy to administer outside hospital such as ECT, or beginning treatment with clozapine;
- detoxification from alcohol or drugs;
- respite care, to give families and other carers a break.

Although each rehabilitation and long-term care service must ensure that it is able to serve each of these functions and look after each group of patients, it may be that some of the functions can be served off the hospital site, or can even be provided by someone other than the health service. For example, respite care with the purpose of giving carers a break could be provided in a hostel set up for that purpose alone, or by extra beds in a hostel which also has long-stay residents. It is those admissions where the patient needs containment in order to be made safe and those for the administration of a specific medical treatment which most obviously require specifically hospital beds.

The deinstitutionalization movement, and the NHS and Community Care Act (Department of Health, 1990), have forced service providers to think about functions rather than places. The danger is that the important functions which the psychiatric institutions served will not be reprovided adequately or appropriately. The challenge is to provide co-ordinated services which are dispersed geographically.

Shepherd (1991) has outlined the advantages of dispersed and centralized models of service provision. He says dispersed models have the following potential advantages:

- smaller units
- greater individualization of care
- greater non-professional involvement
- less institutionalization
- greater integration
- less stigma

but also the following potential disadvantages:

- high initial capital costs
- community resistance
- ghetto-ization
- high revenue costs (staff training and support)
- variability in standards
- isolation.

On the other hand, centralized models, i.e. those based on existing hospitals, have the following potential advantages:

- lower initial capital costs
- economies of scale
- an existing pool of experienced and committed staff
- fewer problems with training and support
- community acceptance;

but also the following potential disadvantages:

- stigma
- loss of individuality
- perpetuation of traditional institutional care practices
- poor community integration.

There are several examples of both models. Time will tell which will prove to be the most effective, although in practice the answer is unlikely to be so clear-cut.

REFERENCES

Bachrach, L. (1980) Overview: model programmes for chronic mental patients. *American Journal of Psychiatry*, **137**(9), 1023–1031.

Bennett, D.H., Folkard, S. and Nicholson, A.K. (1961) Resettlement unit in a mental hospital. *Lancet*, **ii**, 539–541.

Carson, J. and Shaw, L. (1989) Which patients first: a study from the closure of a large psychiatric hospital. *Health Trends*, **21**, 117–120.

Clifford, P., Charman, A., Webb, Y. *et al.* (1991a) Planning for community care: the Community Placement Questionnaire. *British Journal of Clinical Psychology*, **30**, 193–211.

Clifford, P., Charman, A., Webb, Y. and Best, S. (1991b) Planning for community care: long-stay populations of hospitals scheduled for rundown or closure. *British Journal of Psychiatry*, **158**, 190–196.

Creighton, F.J., Hyde, C.E. and Farragher, B. (1991) Douglas House: seven years' experience of a community hostel ward. *British Journal of Psychiatry*, **159**, 500–504.

Dayson, D. and Gooch, C. (1991) *Is Reprovision Impossible for Some Patients?* Paper given at the Sixth Annual Conference of the Team for the Assessment of Psychiatric Services, London, July 1991.

Department of Health, 1990. *National Health Service and Community Care Act*, HMSO, London.

Fryers, T. and Wooff, K. (1989) A decade of mental health care in an English urban community: patterns and trends in Salford, 1976–87, in *Health Service Planning and Research: Contributions from Psychiatric Case Registers*, (ed. J.K. Wing), Gaskell, London.

Garety, P.A., Afele, H.K. and Isaacs, A.D. (1988) A hostel ward for new long-stay psychiatric patients. *Bulletin of the Royal College of Psychiatrists*, **12**, 183–186.

124   Resettlement

Gibbons, J. (1986) Care of 'new' long-stay patients in a District General Hospital Psychiatric Unit: the first two years of a hospital-hostel. *Acta Psychiatrica Scandinavica*, **73**, 582–588.

Goldberg, D.P., Bridges, K., Cooper, W. *et al.* (1985) Douglas House: a new type of hostel ward for chronic psychotic patients. *British Journal of Psychiatry*, **147**, 383–388.

Gudeman, J.E. and Shore, M.F. (1984) Beyond deinstitutionalisation – a new class of facilities for the mentally ill. *New England Journal of Medicine*, **31**(13), 832–836.

Kingdon, D., Turkington, D., Malcolm, K. *et al.* (1991) Replacing the mental hospital. Community provision for a district's chronically psychiatrically disabled in domestic environments? *British Journal of Psychiatry*, **158**, 113–117.

Lawrence, R.E., Copas, J.B. and Cooper, P.W. (1991) Community care: does it reduce the need for psychiatric beds? A comparison of two different styles of service in three hospitals. *British Journal of Psychiatry*, **159**, 334–340.

O'Driscoll, C., Marshall, J. and Reed, J. (1990) Chronically ill psychiatric patients in a District General Hospital Unit: a survey and two-year follow-up in an iner-London Health District. *British Journal of Psychiatry*, **157**, 694–702.

Rowland, L., Perkins, R. and Bennett, D. (1987) Planning community services for the long-term disabled: the Maudsley experience. Unpublished manuscript.

Shepherd, G. (1991) Rehabilitation. Paper given at St George's Hospital, London, 2 November 1991.

Talbott, J.A. and Glick, I.D. (1986) The in-patient care of the chronically mentally ill. *Schizophrenia Bulletin*, **12**, 129–141.

Thornicroft, G. and Bebbington, P. (1899) Deinstitutionalisation – from hospital closure to service development. *British Journal of Psychiatry*, **155**, 739–753.

Thornicroft, G. and Gooch, C. (1991) *Readmission After Discharge – What Are the Risks?* Paper given at the Sixth Annual Conference of the Team for the Assessment of Psychiatric Services, London, July 1991.

Wing, J.K. and Furlong, R. (1986) A haven for the severely disabled within the context of a comprehensive psychiatric community service. *British Journal of Psychiatry*, **149**, 449–457.

Wykes, T. (1982) A hostel-ward for 'new' long-stay patients, in *Long-Term Community Care*, (ed. J.K. Wing). Psychological Medicine, Supplement 2, p. 41–55, Cambridge University Press, Cambridge.

Wykes, T. and Dunn, G. (1992) Cognitive deficit and prediction of rehabilitation success in a chronic psychiatric group. *Psychological Medicine*, **22**, 389–398.

The organization of rehabilitation services

7

Rehabilitation services share the common aim of providing for people with long-term severe psychiatric disability, regardless of whether they live in community settings or in hospital environments. A service's provision includes the identification and the assessment of the needs of its population and it comprises a variety of components for the delivery of treatment and care packages according to fluctuating needs as well as management approaches which ensure integration and continuity (Wing, 1987). Needs can be grouped, for this purpose, into three representative areas of everyday life: occupational, residential and recreational (Wing and Furlong, 1986).

7.1 SERVICE COMPONENTS

Various patterns exist in the way rehabilitation services and their components are structured and organized; these are often based on historical factors and on demographic, political and financial considerations. To a lesser or greater extent, they are also governed by the degree of emphasis each service places on preferred philosophical models. However, information gathered from 18 European rehabilitation services showed that they had seven elements in common: assessment systems, treatment, multidisciplinary work and co-ordination, patient and family involvement in the programme, chains of occupational and residential facilities, continuing support arrangements and some form of service evaluation (Ekdawi, 1990; Rowland, Zeelan and Waismann, 1992). Similarly, experience from the USA showed the essential components of the rehabilitation process to be functional assessments, client involvement, individual rehabilitation planning, direct teaching of skills, assessment and modification of the environment and evaluation of the results, follow-up and consumer involvement in policy and planning (Anthony, Cohen and Farkas, 1982). Achieving a well-organized and integrated service depends on a cycle of planning – evaluation – planning – re-evaluation – re-planning (Wing, 1989).

7.1.1 PLANNING INDIVIDUAL PROGRAMMES

Planning rehabilitation programmes for individuals is based on pooled assessments of their disabilities, their strengths and their needs, as in the model suggested in case presentations (Chapter 3).

7.1.2 SERVICE PLANNING

In essence, planning is a research activity; since rehabilitation services rely on multidisciplinary work, this activity has to be carried out jointly by several representative professionals assisted by the users of the service. Planning has to be carried out at several different levels, some of which will be discussed below.

(a) Population needs

Determining population needs starts with an epidemiological overview. It has been shown that, although the incidence of severe psychiatric disorders tends to be similar in different geographical areas, levels of disability vary and are associated with the prevalence of social isolation (Odegaard, 1953; Sainsbury, 1955) as well as with social deprivation (Jarman, 1983; Thornicroft, Margolius and Jones, 1992). Although regional variations have always to be taken into account (Alanen *et al.*, 1989), these variations are not constant over time; Der (1989), for instance, advises caution in interpreting statistics and point prevalence because of fluctuations in population size and characteristics and the variations in population mobility rates.

Both quantitative and qualitative methods are used to establish a population base from which predictions can be made on the levels of provisions needed (Shepherd, 1988). The quantitative method, which relies on statistical information, is limited by the difficulties in assessing the total number of people requiring certain services because of such fluctuations. Moreover, the usual sources of such information are the statistics of contacts with some statutory services, mainly hospital and social services, which often exclude people receiving care from their family doctors as well as those not in contact. Population movements aside, it should also be noted that some groups of patients change in size over time: the accumulation of 'new' long-stay patients is a case in point.

The qualitative method, on the other hand, is based on the views and choices of service users. Despite its obvious importance, it is limited by the fact that many have difficulties in verbal skills and may lack the necessary ability or assertiveness to express opinions – surveys to elicit consumer preferences are often dominated by the views of vocal minorities who are not necessarily representative. Opinions are also changeable, the changes being subject to fluctuating mental state. It is also often the case that choices are prejudiced through ignorance of what options may be available.

Consulting relatives and other carers on the range of provisions is vital, although their views may be diametrically opposed to those of the clients or the staff. Although such differences may well result in compromises having to be made, it is, however, important not to take views and wishes at face value, but to examine them in depth – a common ground may then be found. For example, relatives may strongly express the view that hospital is the best place for the patient. In this case, they may be saying that the hospital's functions of providing shelter, supervision and support are needed, and they may therefore accept alternative living accommodation which provides such functions. Similarly, the opinions of the professional staff may be restricted by what provisions are on offer.

It will therefore be readily seen that each of the two methods used in assessing population needs for planning purposes is an imperfect instrument if used singly; a combination of both methods has a better chance of giving accurate estimates. A satisfactory way would be to combine information from a case register with surveys of users' views.

(b) 'Norms' and facilities

The paper *Better Services for the Mentally Ill* (Department of Health and Social Security, 1975) was a landmark in British psychiatry in that it contained guidance on levels of service provision such as numbers of sheltered housing and day care places. Its importance was eclipsed by later work highlighting the possible variations in population needs so that, 10 years later, it was stated that such precise norms were not adequate and that local circumstances should dictate levels of service (House of Commons, 1985). Discarding 'norms', however, may well be a case of throwing the baby out with the bath water. Service Planning must start from a baseline and, despite their obvious defects stemming from their sweeping generalizations, 'norms' often serve as 'bench-marks or minimum guidelines below which levels of service should not fall and . . . should therefore not be abandoned' (Shepherd, 1988).

Quantitatively, these levels take into account the various facilities to be provided and the range of places available within them. As a baseline, each district's service should comprise rehabilitation day facilities and rehabilitation units where people are prepared for more independent living, as well as provisions for sheltered work and accommodation including continuing care hostels (Richmond Fellowship, 1983). The number of places in a facility could be determined by the quantitative and qualitative specifications of the target population, guided by the 'norms', and planning should be flexible enough to enable adjustments to be made according to the population's changing needs and so that the results of future evaluations can be accommodated.

Rehabilitation facilities should preferably be sited in the geographical centre of the area they serve so that they are accessible to the bulk of their population, and they should be as near as possible to public services such as shops, transport, hospital, etc. (Acharya et al., 1982). They should not be too widely dispersed, so that a hostel resident, for example, can easily reach his sheltered workplace by public transport; if this is difficult to achieve, alternative transport arrangements would need to be made.

It is a sound principle that rehabilitation facilities should be planned and organized according to the 'stairway' model which enables people to move from one environment to another in easy steps (Wing and Furlong, 1986); it is implicit in this model that compromises may have to be made between individual and group programmes. While acknowledging that the needs of each individual are unique, requiring individual rehabilitation programmes, it is inevitable that some grouping would underpin the planning and organization of facilities in the sense that a group may, for instance, require accommodation with 24-hour staff support, while others may manage more independently. There is a critical mass which determines size, and the viability of a facility may well correlate with the number of its users; thus it is neither feasible nor economical to run a sheltered work facility for, say, four people.

(c) Manpower

The manpower structure of a rehabilitation service is based on the premise that its multidisciplinary team is dedicated to people with psychiatric disability. Generic teams with catchment area responsibility are often ill-equipped to deliver adequate rehabilitation services. Their work tends to be demand-led, with acute illness and emergencies being their main priorities; as a consequence, time-consuming and complex rehabilitation problems tend to take second place and continuity of care may be compromised. It is therefore essential that each district maintains a team whose members have the necessary specialized training and expertise, as well as sufficient time devoted to the rehabilitation and continuing care services (Morgan, 1983).

There is a wealth of literature on the composition and functioning of rehabilitation teams and their organization (e.g. Watts and Bennett, 1983; Wing, 1989). In contrast, there is a dearth of information and guidelines on acceptable staffing levels. The Royal College of Psychiatrists (1992) has recommended that each district of about 300 000 population should have a minimum of one full-time consultant psychiatrist with responsibility for rehabilitation; no such accepted guidelines exist in the case of other core professionals (hospital and community nurses, clinical psychologists, occupational therapists and social workers) and there are substantial variations in the staffing levels amongst rehabilitation services, as illustrated by informal surveys in Britain (Ekdawi, 1990). A model suggested by McCreadie (1986) lists 52 different provisions, including staff numbers, widely accepted to be important in rehabilitation; a rehabilitation unit, for example, would have 18 staff members and nine would be required for support services, but no figures are suggested specifically for each profession.

Calculating reasonable manpower levels should not only be based on direct treatment and care functions, but also on essential time required to relate to other psychiatric teams, to mobilize local and voluntary support and to provide education and training, as well as to liaise with other statutory services including education, police, employment, housing and social security (Farkas and Anthony, 1989).

(d) Coordination

The tasks undertaken by a district's rehabilitation service require high levels of co-ordination. This is crucial particularly where services are provided by several, geographically dispersed units and where community services are shared by a number of agencies. The dangers of poor communication, isolation, duplication and inequalities in the quality and quantity of care provided are ever present. These dangers are augmented by the differing ideologies, standards and background of different team members who may also be accountable to diverse employing authorities.

Although case management is said to have developed in order to mitigate the risks of the fragmentation inherent in disperse community services which resulted from de-institutionalization, it should be recognized that the importance of co-ordinating the work of multidisciplinary teams and agencies has been accepted and successfully practised in rehabilitation services for many years (Affleck, 1981; Ekdawi, 1981). In a discussion of the concept and role of case management in long-term mental illness, Thornicroft (1991) summarized its core tasks as being those of case finding, identification and assessment of needs, designing care packages, co-ordinating and monitoring service delivery, evaluating its effectiveness, modifying the care package and repeating the cycle. Some confusion, however, still surrounds the definition and the role of case management (Bachrach, 1989) but, in any case, a system which ensures that agencies pool their resources by setting up multidisciplinary teams whose work is targeted at the needs of people requiring long-term intensive support is the best way forward (Holloway, 1991). The formula of having a principal co-ordinating device whatever form it takes, has stood the test of time as a key element in the organization of rehabilitation services.

A suggested organizational pattern would be to form a 'bottom up' chain of service co-ordination consisting, at least, of four main elements.

- A key worker who would have a long-term therapeutic relationship with the client and his/her carers, and who would be easily contactable by them. The key worker ensures that care programmes (agreed at care programme meetings or case presentations) are implemented and regularly reviewed. The other multidisciplinary rehabilitation team members support the key worker and may potentially undertake some of his/her work.
- The multidisciplinary team whose members carry out the variety of necessary clinical, social and vocational assessments and who provide the treatment and care packages.
- A case manager who negotiates and facilitates the essential resources for assessment and care with the team and other relevant agencies.
- A rehabilitation committee which has a wide membership among representatives of statutory and voluntary organizations as well as of service users. The committee has an overview of the district's rehabilitation service provisions and it investigates its population needs so that it can recommend policies/plan service developments and review progress.

There are many advanges to a team, rather than an individual responsibility and commitment to a 'case'. A key worker or a case manager working more or less in isolation could find it difficult to maintain objectivity and might become disillusioned and suffer 'burn-out'; single individuals are in a weaker negotiating position than a whole team; continuity of care could be severely disrupted if they move away.

REFERENCES

Acharaya, S., Ekdawi, M.Y., Gallagher, L. and Glaister, B. (1982) Day hospital rehabilitation: a six-year study. *Social Psychiatry*, **17**, 1–5.

Affleck, J.W. (1981) The Edinburgh progressive care system, in *Handbook of Psychiatric Rehabilitation Practice*, (eds J.K. Wing and B. Morris), Oxford University Press, Oxford.

Alanen, Y.O., Salokangas, R.K.R., Ojanen, M. *et al.* (1989) Tertiary prevention: treatment and rehabilitation of schizophrenic patients – results of the Finnish National Programme, in *The Public Health Impact of Mental Disorder*, (eds D. Goldberg and D. Tantam), Hogrefe & Huber, Toronto.

Anthony, W.A., Cohen, M.R. and Farkas, M. (1982) A psychiatric rehabilitation program: 'can I recognise one when I see one?' *Community Mental Health Journal*, **18**, 83–95.

Bachrach, L. (1989) Case management: toward a shared definition. *Hospital and Community Psychiatry*, **40**, 883.

Department of Health and Social Security (1975) *Better Services for the Mentally Ill*. Cmnd 6233. HMSO, London.

Der, G. (1989) The effects of population changes on long-stay in-patient rates, in *Health Services Planning and Research: Contributions from Psychiatric Case Registers*. Royal College of Psychiatrists, London.

Ekdawi, M.Y. (1981) Rehabilitation practice at Netherne Hospital, in *Handbook of Psychiatric Rehabilitation Practice*, (eds J.K. Wing and B. Morris), Oxford University Press, Oxford.

Ekdawi, M.Y. (1990) The components of psychiatric rehabilitation services, in *International Perspectives in Schizophrenia*, (ed. M. Weller), John Libbey, London.

Farkas, M. and Anthony, W.A. (eds) (1989) *Psychiatric Rehabilitation Programs: Putting Theory Into Practice*, Johns Hopkins University Press, Baltimore.

Holloway, F. (1991) Case management for the mentally ill: looking at the evidence. *International Journal of Social Psychiatry*, **37**, 2–13.

House of Commons (1985) *Second Report from the Social Services Committee*, HMSO, London.

Jarman, B. (1983) Identification of underprivileged areas. *British Medical Journal*, **286**, 805–812.

McCreadie, R.G. (1986) Rehabilitation, in *Contemporary Issues in Schizophrenia*, (eds A. Kerr and P. Smith), Gaskell, London.

Morgan, R. (1983) Industrial therapy in the mental hospital, in *Theory and Practice of Psychiatric Rehabilitation* (eds F.N. Watts and D.H. Bennett), John Wiley & Sons, Chichester.

Odegaard, O. (1953) New data on marriage and mental disease. *Journal of Mental Science*, **99**, 778–785.

Richmond Fellowship (1983) *Mental Health and the Community: Report of the Richmond Fellowship Enquiry*, Richmond Fellowship Press, London.

Rowland, L.A., Zeelan, J. and Waismann, L.C. (1992) Patterns of service for the long-term mentally ill in Europe. *British Journal of Clinical Psychology*, **31**, 405–417.

Royal College of Psychiatrists (1992) *The Role of a Rehabilitation Consultant in a Psychiatric Service*, Royal College of Psychiatrists, London.

Shepherd, G. (1988) Evaluation of service planning, in *Community Care in Practice,* (eds A. Lavender and F. Holloway), John Wiley & Sons, Chichester.

Sainsbury, P. (1955) *Suicide in London: an Ecological Study,* Maudsley Monograph No. 1, Chapman & Hall, London.

Thornicroft, G. (1991) Case management in long-term mental illness. *International Review of Psychiatry,* **3**, 125–132.

Thornicroft, G., Margolius, O. and Jones, D (1992) The TAPS Project: new long-stay psychiatric patients and social deprivation. *British Journal of Psychiatry,* **161**, 621–624.

Watts, F. and Bennett, D. (1983) Management of the staff team, in *Theory and Practice of Psychiatric Rehabilitation* (eds F. Watts and D.H. Bennett), John Wiley & Sons, Chichester.

Wing, J.K. (1987) Medical and social sciences and medical and social care, in *Social Care and Research,* (eds J. Barnes and N. Connelly), Bedford Square Press, London.

Wing, J.K. (1989) Planning services for long-term psychiatric disorder, in *The Public Health Impact of Mental Disorder,* (eds D. Goldberg and D. Tantam), Hogrefe & Huber, Toronto.

Wing, J.K. and Furlong, R. (1986) A haven for the severely disabled within the context of a comprehensive psychiatric community service. *British Journal of Psychiatry,* **149**, 449–457.

Rehabilitation outcomes 8

Rehabilitation services are founded on the assumption that their programmes and interventions result in positive effects on the outcome of
long-term disorders (Dion and Anthony, 1987) and their *raison d'être*,
therefore, is that they are able to achieve significant changes in the health
and social functioning of their target groups. These changes, or outcomes, should be both measurable and reproducible so that useful and
successful models and practices are identified; this, in turn, would point
the way to improvements in the quality of services provided and would
prompt future research. In addition, outcome measurements are
required to satisfy policy and funding authorities; with the mounting
emphasis on reducing health care costs, there is continuing pressure
on all medical services and rehabilitation programmes to produce outcome data (Wagner, 1987). In order to contain expenditure, there is an
increasing drive to prioritize resource allocation and to develop systems
of ranking services according to their efficiency in reducing mortality
and morbidity. Inevitably, the survival of services which are labour-
intensive and time-consuming, which target disorders of uncertain
aetiology and long-term course, and whose outcome results may be
inconclusive, could be threatened. It is therefore necessary to examine
some of the salient problems of choosing and implementing methods
of quality assurance and auditing of rehabilitation outcomes.

8.1 WHAT IS TO BE MEASURED

In reviewing a number of scientific studies on the long-term outcome
of schizophrenia, for example, Wing (1988) asserted that, among the
technical issues involved, two clinical problems were pre-eminent:
how schizophrenia is to be defined and what is meant by outcome;
generalizability of results is dependent on the extent to which
diagnostic and outcome criteria are reproducible. He concluded that
we are still far from achieving such comparability. These dilemmas
become even more daunting in rehabilitation, since the services

provide for assorted disorders (although schizophrenia may form a significant proportion) with diverse, fluctuating courses and where diagnosis is made with varying degrees of confidence. Moreover, as Fuhrer (1987) pointed out, a rehabilitation outcome is never directly observed; improvements in self-care skills or employability, for example, can only be deemed to be rehabilitation outcomes if we infer that these changes are a direct result of services delivered. Many observable changes, in the long term, could be due to a variety of factors not necessarily related to the rehabilitation interventions.

8.2 INTERPRETATION OF RESULTS

Decisions on what is to be measured in auditing outcome are liable to pose problems, being dependent on a multitude of factors including the philosophy and the theoretical framework of the auditors, as well as on their value systems, beliefs and professional and social class backgrounds. Definitions of quality of care, for example, vary in emphasis between behaviour therapists, psychoanalysts and 'normalizers', and measurements may be based on assumptions about what is perceived as desirable rather than on established empirical relationships (Shepherd, 1988). Outcome results may be interpreted differently by different professionals. For instance, the fact that a man with an unusual sexual orientation has ceased to engage in activities that previously resulted in offending behaviour may be regarded by a behaviourist to be a successful outcome. This may not, however, be perceived in the same way by a psychoanalyst if the underlying causes of these activities still persisted. Some outcomes, including improved earning capacity and reduction in unemployment are understandable and valued by the general public; others, such as work satisfaction and increased activities and friendships, which present difficulties in measurement, may be less so (Farkas and Anthony, 1987).

8.2.1 INDIVIDUAL OUTCOMES

The question 'what does rehabilitation accomplish?' was asked in a discussion paper by Strauss (1986); he challenged the assumption that all rehabilitation does is to compensate for deficits which are seen as largely immutable, since advances in knowledge suggest that, in severe disorders such as schizophrenia, rehabilitation is not just a palliative which compensates for deficits, but may actually contribute to the process of recovery. Strauss also pointed out that research has often neglected to focus on the impact of rehabilitation on the individual's personal aspects, including his/her sense of identity. Although managing and compensating for handicap is an important rehabilitation goal, rehabilitation also aims at reducing symptoms and symptomatic behaviour and at preventing further disability.

Rehabilitation can also effect measurable improvement by enhancing self-esteem and confidence and significantly altering the rehabilitee's self-concept. This was reported, for example, by Wing (1966) in a rehabilitation unit where self-confidence in the face of severe disablement was both valued and attainable. In a three-year follow up study (Collis and Ekdawi, 1987), rehabilitation outcomes included a gradual rejection by the rehabilitees of the patient role and increased levels of self-esteem and feelings of well-being and normality; they were less likely to see their illness as a burden and to view the hospital as a refuge and they also expanded their non-hospital contacts. Additional detailed measurements in the same group (Collis, 1986) demonstrated changes in their sense of identity; they felt subjectively better and they showed a substantial shift towards a more positive self-concept. The majority viewed their real self as being normal compared with 'most psychiatric patients'. There is therefore no realistic basis to the pessimistic view that rehabilitation is just a damage-limitation exercise; it can accomplish fundamental changes on a personal level. It is therefore important to include measures, such as those of attitudes and self-confidence, as rehabilitation outcome indicators.

8.2.2 SERVICE OUTCOMES

Two main questions have to be addressed in evaluating a rehabilitation service's outcomes: what does the service set out to achieve in relation to the needs of its population and how far has it achieved it? The starting point is to define, as clearly as possible, the expressed aims of the service in meeting assessed needs; thus the aims may be to improve work competence and domestic functioning within certain environments and to reduce the incidence of suicidal attempts. Declarations of vague, non-specific intentions, such as improving independence, should be avoided. Achieving the aims presupposes that the service has adequate provisions in terms of physical plant, suitable manpower and administrative support, that its practices conform to criteria indicative of acceptable care and that its patients/clients have consistently complied with agreed programmes (Donabedian, 1966).

8.3 THE RATIONALE OF SOME COMMONLY USED OUTCOME MEASURES

Outcome can be measured in terms of the impact of rehabilitation interventions, such as skills training, drug therapy and community support, on the individual's clinical state and social performance. Farkas and Anthony (1987) enumerated the shortcomings of many of the outcome studies: there is a dearth of studies which employ designs that permit reasonable causal inferences to be made; many have used post-test only designs, and non-random assignment designs are common; the populations studied are heterogeneous and follow-up periods are too brief. There is often lack of specificity, and hence poor replicability, of treatment approaches as well as lack of reliable and valid measures. Some of the deficiencies are difficult to rectify; many services, for example, are not in a position to exercise very strict population selection criteria and random assignment designs may raise ethical issues.

With these reservations in mind, many rehabilitation services have measured their outcomes by means of certain 'hard' data, mainly hospital admission rates and employment status on follow-up; this is illustrated by the longitudinal Netherne studies (Ekdawi, 1972; Acharya et al., 1982) and the large scale Toronto study (Goering et al. 1982). Such measures have the advantage that the data are usually readily available and easily objectified and understood, allowing comparison. Other studies have used standardized instruments to assess changes in the mental state and social performance of fairly homogeneous populations over time (Lavender, 1987; Hyde et al., 1987). Such studies are of outstanding interest, but they also raise complex issues in relating outcomes to interventions.

Hospital admissions.   The number and frequency of hospital admissions, as well as the duration of periods of hospitalization, have been extensively used as outcome indicators. Hospitalization, however, should not be taken at face value as denoting failure of rehabilitation. Local policies and individual clinical judgements often dictate the threshold at which the decision to admit to hospital is made; it is also conditional on the availability of hospital beds and of alternative residential places and community support. In some cases, the purpose of planned hospital admissions is to provide respite and to forestall crises and they may therefore indicate a positive rather than a negative outcome; in analysing hospitalization data, therefore, a method of differentiating such admissions from those generated by symptom relapse has to be agreed.

Employment status.   Employment has been recognized as a meaningful outcome measure since it implies reduced dependency and a good level of social adjustment, provided it is of reasonable duration (6 or 9 months in any one job). Alternatively, periods of unemployment have served as an acceptable indicator. However, employment status does not necessarily correlate with employability as it is highly dependent on prevalent economic and political factors and it can therefore give a distorted picture of a service's performance. A more reliable, though more complex, indicator is the ability of its rehabilitees to acquire and maintain a work role and to engage in constructive work activity in the environments which best suit them.

Clinical state.   Improved mental state, symptom control and reduced incidence of suicidal behaviour are related to compliance with medication, levels and quality of available support systems and constructive daytime occupation; they reflect, to a large extent, the overall performance of the service. Nevertheless, some environmental influences and life events, as well as less specific factors such as natural remissions in the course of illness, should be taken into account. Care must therefore be exercised in relating long-term changes in the mental state, particularly those which influence behaviour and community adaptation, to specific rehabilitation interventions.

Social performance.   The levels of social adjustment attained and their stability have served as important rehabilitation outcome indicators, because of their effects on community tenure and since they dictate the type and amount of professional input. As in the case of clinical state assessments, however, the multitude of contributory factors may be difficult to tease out and, consequently, establishing cause and effect may not be possible.

The use of combinations of standardized instruments, over a period of several years, to measure changes in rehabilitees' mental state and social functioning and to relating them to rates of hospitalization and of engagement in work activities have formed an appropriate basis for the measurement of rehabilitation outcomes. Adopting such measures and applying them in a variety of rehabilitation settings (Farkas and Anthony, 1989) is the only way towards more accurate and generalizable outcome criteria, but it should be borne in mind that, in the current state of knowledge, these are still crude, imperfect measures which give rise to as many questions as answers and that their results should always be cautiously interpreted. Finally, the positive influences of rehabilitation on an individual level, such as changes in attitudes and in the perception of self-identity, should be included in the measurement outcome.

REFERENCES

Acharya, S., Ekdawi, M.Y., Gallagher, L. and Glaister, B. (1982) Day hospital rehabilitation: a six-year study. *Social Psychiatry*, **17**, 1–5.

Collis, M. (1986) *The Self Concept in Psychiatric rehabilitation*. University of Surrey. PhD Thesis.

Collis, M. and Ekdawi, M.Y. (1984) Social adjustment in rehabilitation. *International Journal of Rehabilitation Research*, **7**, 259–272.

Donabedian, A. (1966) Evaluating the quality of medical care. *Milbank Memorial Fund Quarterly*, **44**, 166–206.

Dion, G.L. and Anthony, W.A. (1987) Research in psychiatric rehabilitation: a review of experimental and quasi-experimental studies. *Rehabilitation Counselling Bulletin*, **3**, 177–203.

Ekdawi, M.Y. (1972) The Netherne Resettlement Unit: results of ten years. *British Journal of Psychiatry*, **121**, 417–27.

Farkas, M. and Anthony, W.A. (1987) Outcome analysis in psychiatric rehabilitation, in *Rehabilitation Outcomes: Analysis and Measurement*, (ed. M.J. Fuhrer), Brookes Publishing, Baltimore.

Fuhrer, M.J. (1987) Overview of outcome analysis in rehabilitation, in *Rehabilitation Outcomes: Analysis and Measurement*, (ed. M.J. Fuhrer), Paul H. Brookes, Baltimore.

Goering, P., Wasylenki, D., Lance, W. and Freeman, S.J.J. (1982) From hospital to community. *Journal of Nervous and Mental Disease*, **172**, 667–673.

Hyde, C., Bridges, K., Goldberg, D. *et al.* (1987) The evaluation of a hostel ward – a controlled study using cost-benefit analysis. *British Journal of Psychiatry*, **151**, 805–812.

Lavender, A. (1987) Improving the quality of care on psychiatric rehabilitation wards: a controlled evaluation. *British Journal of Psychiatry*, **150**, 476–481.

Shepherd, G. (1988) Evaluation of service planning, in *Community Care in Practice*, (eds A. Lavender and F. Holloway), John Wiley & Sons, Chichester.

Strauss, J.S. (1986) Discussion: What does rehabilitation accomplish? *Schizophrenia Bulletin*, **12**, 720–723.

Wagner, K.A. (1987) Outcome analysis in comprehensive medical rehabilitation, in *Rehabilitation Outcomes: Analysis and Measurement*, (ed. M.J. Fuhrer), Brookes Publishing, Baltimore.

Wing, J.K. (1988) Comments on the long-term outcome of schizophrenia. *Schizophrenia Bulletin*, **14**, 669–675.

Index